COMPREHENSIVE MANAGEMENT
of
Hemophilia

COMPREHENSIVE MANAGEMENT
of
Hemophilia

Editor

DONNA C. BOONE, R.P.T.

Research Coordinator
Orthopaedic Hospital
Los Angeles, California

F. A. DAVIS COMPANY, PHILADELPHIA

Library of Congress Cataloging in Publication Data
Main entry under title:

Comprehensive management of hemophilia.

  Includes bibliographical references and index.
  1. Hemophilia.   2. Hemophilia—Complications and
sequelae.   I. Boone, Donna C., 1932-
RC642.C64   616.1'57   76-18109
ISBN 0-8036-1000-9

Dedicated To

CHARLES LEROY LOWMAN, M.D.

Founder of Orthopaedic Hospital

and

Pioneer of Many Concepts

of Total Patient Care

FOREWORD

The modern era of blood coagulation began in the 1940s when many unknown pro-coagulants of the blood were recognized. *Pari passu* the basic clotting defect in hemophilia was defined. Aided by the availability of hemophilic animals, accurate diagnosis and a rational basis for the management of hemorrhage with transfusion therapy became a reality. Thus, the frustrating plight of the hemophiliac was radically changed to one of hope and a near normal life by what amounted to a major breakthrough in one aspect of medical care. First of these advances in treatment was the use of fresh frozen plasma, frequently and intensively administered in controlling hemorrhage. The advent of cryoprecipitates and higher potency plasma concentrates made normalization of hemostasis in the hemophiliac feasible for days and even weeks and longer. With this, many medical procedures which had previously been life threatening and even fatal, such as tooth extraction and surgery, became commonplace and no more complicated than in individuals without a hemorrhagic disorder.

The translation of scientific advances into effective diagnostic and management programs is the aim of all medical research. In no area have the practical rewards from research been greater than in the hemophilia field. While the affected individual often bemoans the lag time which occurs in this translational effort, in actuality the elapsed time from discovery to application in the hemophilia field has been remarkably short. A major effort in mobilizing the health resources of a community is essential, however, if the application of newer knowledge is to be effective. The costs may be great, but the benefits are greater.

No area in the United States, or probably anywhere, has done a better job in marshalling the necessary medical and social resources required to cope with the management problems of hemophilia than in the Los Angeles, California area. It is a tribute to the vision of the staff of the Orthopaedic Hospital that they recognized the need to assemble in one center members of the various disciplines required for the effective treatment and rehabilitation of the community's hemophiliacs; included are the disciplines of hematology, clinical pathology, orthopedics, pediatrics, psychiatry, dentistry, nursing, physical therapy, psychology, vocational guidance, and social work.

This book provides an excellent guide to the practical applications of modern science and medicine in all its aspects in the hemophilia field today. The hemophilia center at Los Angeles is a prototype of community organization in the delivery of specialized health care services and can provide a guiding light for other communities in the mobilization of health manpower. Essential in this undertaking is the education of hemophiliacs and their families in how best to take advantage of the mobilized resources and to minimize what might otherwise be adverse effects of the disease. The cooperation of hemophilia centers and voluntary health organizations as represented by the National Hemophilia Foundation and the World Federation of Hemophilia can be of great aid in the development of new centers and their utilization. This book should also provide an example to the medical, dental and allied health professions, as well as to health care planners, legislators, and others who should be jointly responsible for the developing new order in medical care, of how a chronic disease problem may be effectively approached once the basic knowledge for management has been developed.

K. M. Brinkhous, M.D.
Alumni Distinguished Professor of Pathology
University of North Carolina at Chapel Hill

FOREWORD

This book is proof of the superb services offered by the Los Angeles Hemophilia Rehabilitation Center. These services were envisioned by the late Dr. Madeleine Fallon, the first medical director, and Alfred R. Dubin, then President of the Hemophilia Foundation of Southern California, when they initiated and supported the establishment of a Center at Orthopaedic Hospital over a decade ago. Through comprehensive therapy covering every facet of this complicated genetic disorder, exemplary control of the disease became possible. Indeed, the Los Angeles Center attracts many patients from all over the country and enjoys international recognition.

In close consultations with the prudent managers of the Center, we were able to stimulate the enactment of satisfactory legislation in California. This Hemophilia bill, which is the most comprehensive in the United States to date, provides coverage including home treatment, prophylactic therapy, and corrective surgery for all hemophiliacs.

We feel privileged to financially support the publication of this book just as we have funded services for patients, research activities, and other educational materials.

Comprehensive Management of Hemophilia will promote the continuation of excellent services at this Center and will guide other institutions in the development of similar services, all directed toward the ultimate objective of perfecting control of this disease. We are confident that we are playing an effective role in the maintenance and expansion of this program.

Walter Platz, Ph.D.
Executive Director
Hemophilia Foundation of
Southern California

PREFACE

"To heal even an eye, one must heal the head, and indeed the whole body."

(Hippocrates)

This book represents the culmination of 12 years' experience in the comprehensive management of the varied manifestations of hemophilia. Contributions are multi-disciplined and reflect the particular philosophy of rehabilitation conceptualized at the Hemophilia Rehabilitation Center at Orthopaedic Hospital, Los Angeles, California. Hematologic developments during the past decade have produced marked changes in the effectiveness of medical care and have had even greater impact upon the lives of those persons with hemophilia. Indeed, these developments have permitted rehabilitative advances which were only dreams a decade ago.

Progress has been made in the third chapter in the history of hemophilia, as described by C. B. Kerr,* with the temporary normalization of the disturbed coagulation status of the hemophiliac. Hopefully, during the next decade this chapter will be completed with control or permanent suppression of these disorders and their medical, psychological, and social ramifications.

Donna C. Boone

---

*Kerr, C. B.: The Fortunes of Haemophiliacs in the Nineteenth Century. *Medical History*, 7 (4): 359, (Oct) 1963.

ACKNOWLEDGEMENTS

My gratitude is offered to Walter Platz, Ph.D., Executive Director, and the officers and Board of Directors of the Hemophilia Foundation of Southern California for their generous support of the publication of this book as well as their continued interest and encouragement.

I wish to thank all the contributors to this book. Additionally, many other people contribute in many ways to the day-to-day patient care and functioning of the Hemophilia Rehabilitation Center. Shirley Whiteman, M.D., pediatrician and Carol Spence, R.P.T., physical therapist, continue to serve the Center and its patients with expertise as do all the physical therapists and nurses who provide on-going treatment for the large number of hemophilic patients who receive care at this Center. Thanks are also extended to Mary Ann Pattinson, M.A., educational and vocational counselor; and to Audrey Parks and Debbie Williams who manage clerical and secretarial activities.

Former staff members of the Center currently pursuing other endeavors but remembered fondly for their past contributions include: Max Negri, M.D., orthopedic surgeon; Osamu Chiono, D.D.S., pedodontist; Phillip Weise, Ph.D., psychologist; JoAnn Parham, R.P.T., physical therapist; Flora Franklin, P.H.N., public health nurse; J. Douglas McDonald, coagulation laboratory technician; Florence Cromwell, O.T.R., occupational therapist; Jackie Godokiss, R.N., emergency room nursing supervisor; Mary Bonilla, R.N., intravenous administration nurse; Wayne Edwards, M.S., rehabilitation counselor; James Holt, Ph.D., research consultant; George Crisp, M.D., internist; Jerome Franklin, M.D., psychiatrist; Dunham Gilbert, Ph.D., research statistician; Eleanor Frank and Janice Woo Chin, secretarial staff.

The continued support of James Heidenreich, Executive Administrator, the administrative and medical staffs, and the Board of Trustees of Orthopaedic Hospital has permitted the Center to grow and expand; special gratitude is expressed to Mary F. Thweatt, former Hospital Director, and the late Lee Sanders, Hospital Executive Vice President, as well as to William Stryker, M.D. and J. Vernon Luck, M.D., past Medical Directors.

The late Andon A. Andonian, M.D., internist, and Madeleine Fallon, M.D., hematologist, are remembered with affection for their dedicated care and concern for hemophilic patients and for their many years of service to the Hemophilia Foundation of Southern California.

Special tribute is accorded to Annabel Anabel for her work on the preliminary manuscripts as well as for her constant moral support and to Ann Lowe for typing final manuscript.

Lastly, a thank you to all our patients for their cooperation and countenance.

CONTRIBUTORS

ALFRED BENJAMIN, R.B.P., Chief Medical Photographer, Orthopaedic Hospital, Los Angeles, California.

ENID F. ECKERT, R.N., Outpatient Nurse, Hemophilia Rehabilitation Center, Orthopaedic Hospital, Los Angeles, California.

DONNA C. BOONE, R.P.T., Research Coordinator and Research Physical Therapist, Hemophilia Rehabilitation Center, Orthopaedic Hospital, Los Angeles, California.

SHELBY L. DIETRICH, M.D., Director, Hemophilia Rehabilitation Center, Orthopaedic Hospital, and Associate Clinical Professor, School of Medicine, University of Southern California, Los Angeles, California.

CHARLES H. HURT, M.S.W., Psychiatric Social Worker, Hemophilia Rehabilitation Center, Orthopaedic Hospital, Los Angeles, California.

CAROL K. KASPER, M.D., Hematologist, Hemophilia Rehabilitation Center, Orthopaedic Hospital, and Associate Professor, School of Medicine, University of Southern California, Los Angeles, California.

ALICE MARTINSON, M.D., Orthopaedic Surgeon, Hemophilia Rehabilitation Center, Orthopaedic Hospital, Los Angeles, California and Chief, Orthopaedic Surgery, Naval Regional Medical Center, Long Beach, California.

THOMAS F. MULKEY, D.D.S., Oral Surgeon, Hemophilia Rehabilitation Center, Orthopaedic Hospital, and Assistant Clinical Professor of Oral Surgery, School of Dentistry, University of Southern California, Los Angeles, California.

DAVID POWELL, D.D.S., M.S., Pedodontist, Hemophilia Rehabilitation Center, Orthopaedic Hospital, and Director of Training for Dentistry, University Affiliated Project, Children's Hospital, Los Angeles, California.

JORDAN RHODES, M.D., former Orthopaedic Surgeon, Hemophilia Rehabilitation Center, Orthopaedic Hospital, Los Angeles, California.

RICHARD R. SCHREIBER, M.D., Radiologist, Orthopaedic Hospital, and Assistant Clinical Professor of Radiology, School of Medicine, University of Southern California, Los Angeles, California.

CHARLOTTE TAYLOR, M.S., former Rehabilitation Counselor, Hemophilia Rehabilitation Center, Orthopaedic Hospital; Coordinator of Research and Training, Medical Rehabilitation Research and Training Center, and Assistant Clinical Professor of Rehabilitative Medicine, School of Medicine, University of Southern California, Los Angeles, California.

NANCY TAYLOR, Financial Coordinator, Hemophilia Rehabilitation Center, Orthopaedic Hospital, Los Angeles, California.

CONTENTS

1

INTRODUCTION

Donna C. Boone

The Hemophilia Rehabilitation Center at Orthopaedic Hospital, Los Angeles, had its beginnings in 1962 when the Hemophilia Foundation of Southern California contracted with the hospital for the provision of inpatient and outpatient services for Foundation members. Since its organization in 1951, the Foundation has been intimately involved in the struggle for provision of adequate care for hemophilic patients in the Southern California area and in the problems of financing such care.

The Center was funded through two grants from the Department of Health, Education, and Welfare for the period 1964 through June 1970. The funding initially supported a Hemophilia Demonstration Project; when this Project terminated, support was granted for a Regional Hemophilia Rehabilitation Center. Since 1970 the Center has been supported through fees for patient services and contributions from the Hemophilia Foundation of Southern California and from Orthopaedic Hospital.

From the beginning, the Center staff has been multidisciplinary in scope; the Hemophilia Demonstration Project represented a "first" in hemophilic rehabilitation since it combined in one coordinated setting all the professional specialists required to diagnose and to treat the multiple problems manifested by this disease. Comprehensive medical, psychosocial, and vocational-educational services are offered by the staff composed of a Center Director who serves also as Center pediatrician, another pediatrician, an internist, a hematologist, a coagulation laboratory technician, an orthopedist, two outpatient nurses, a clinical physical therapist, a research physical therapist, a pedodontist, an oral surgeon, a psychiatric social worker, a vocational rehabilitation counselor, and a photographer. Psychiatric and other consultants are available.

The objectives of the Center are to offer to the individual with hemophilia the opportunity for adequate diagnostic, treatment, and long-term rehabilitation services; to stimulate education and research into the various aspects of this disease; and to serve as a resource to aid other institutions in developing local treatment and rehabilitation services. International recognition was extended to the Center in 1970 when it was designated as an International Training Center by the World Federation of Hemophilia.

Although the Center was established originally to serve patients living in the southwestern United States, increasing numbers of patients come from throughout the United States, and Central and South America for short-term evaluation and/or long-term rehabilitation. Registered patients numbered 182 in 1964, 263 in 1967, 598 in 1973, and 647 in 1975. Of this latter figure, approximately 350 to 400 patients are actively treated persons who depend on this Center for their total care. Seventy-five percent have hemophilia A, 20 percent have hemophilia B, and the remaining 5 percent have von Willebrand's disease and other coagulation defects. The age distribution of the patient group reflects increased longevity since 57 percent of the group is over 20 years of age.

Midway through the life of the Center, Factor VIII concentrates and cryoprecipitate and Factor IX concentrate replaced fresh frozen or lyophilized plasma as therapeutic products of choice. Increased availability of these products permitted greater emphasis on outpatient rather than inpatient management and allowed major surgical procedures to be performed without undue risk under hematologic supervision.

Certain concepts developed during the initial and middle phases of the existence of the Center continue to be valid today even though the hematologic control of the disease has changed markedly. Final reports from the two grant periods, *Hemophilia: A Total Approach to Treatment and Rehabilitation* and *Hemophilia and the Regional Center Concept*, provide complete information about the Center during its various stages of development. These documents, available at Orthopaedic Hospital, are particularly helpful to institutions in the embryonic development of a hemophilic rehabilitation center. One concept developed and nurtured during the Center's formative years deserves special emphasis: the complex problems of hemophilia can best be managed in a coordinated setting with adequate medical care combined with all the services of the rehabilitation specialties.

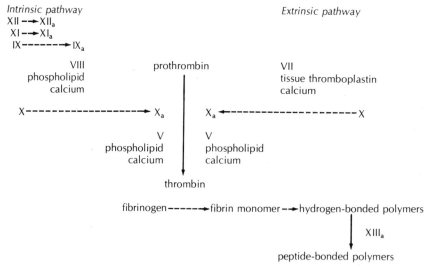

Figure 2-1. Interaction of clotting factors

2

HEMATOLOGIC CARE

Carol K. Kasper

NORMAL HEMOSTASIS

When a blood vessel is severed, hemostasis is achieved by a sequence of events. The vessel constricts, thus limiting the outflow of blood. Platelets adhere to the exposed subendothelial connective tissue and aggregate, forming a soft platelet plug which may suffice in smaller vessels. In the stagnant blood proximal to the platelet plug in the vessel, plasma clotting factors and phospholipid, released from the aggregated platelets, interact to convert fibrinogen to fibrin monomer. The monomers polymerize into fibrin strands, which enmesh the blood cells to form the familiar red clot. The reactions of the plasma clotting factors and the formation of a stable fibrin network will be discussed below.

Nomenclature

The International Committee on Thrombosis and Haemostasis assigned roman numerals to the plasma clotting factors and arabic numerals to platelet substances involved in coagulation. The terms Factor I, Factor II, Factor III and Factor IV are rarely used since the familiar names are preferred. There is no Factor VI; the number was used to describe a substance now recognized to be only an intermediate in the clotting sequence. The other plasma clotting factors are described by their roman numeral designations in common parlance. Some of the clotting factors are activated during clotting; the activated form of a clotting factor is designated by the subscript$_a$, for example, activated Factor X is written X_a.

The following is a list of the International and the familiar names of the clotting factors:

International Name	Familiar Name(s)
Factor I	Fibrinogen
Factor II	Prothrombin
Factor III	Tissue thrombo-plastin
Factor IV	Calcium
Factor V	Proaccelerin, labile factor
Factor VII	Proconvertin, stable factor
Factor VIII	Antihemophilic factor (AHF), anti-hemophilic globulin (AHG)
Factor IX	Plasma thrombo-plastin com-ponent (PTC), Christmas factor
Factor X	Stuart-Prower factor
Factor XI	Plasma thrombo-plastin antece-dent (PTA)
Factor XII	Hageman factor
Factor XIII	Fibrin stabilizing factor, Laki-Lorand factor

Current Understanding of the Interaction of Clotting Factors

There are two pathways, namely, the extrinsic and the intrinsic, by which clotting factors may interact to generate thrombin, and thereby cause the formation of fibrin (Fig. 2-1).

In the *extrinsic pathway*, Factor VII acts as an enzyme catalyzing the interaction of tissue thromboplastin (a lipoprotein

3

found in the tissues, especially in brain, lung, and placenta) and calcium with Factor X to form Factor X_a. Then, in a manner not yet clearly understood, Factor X_a, Factor V, phospholipid from platelets (platelet factor 3), and calcium form a complex which converts prothrombin to thrombin. Thrombin splits two pairs of peptides from fibrinogen, leaving fibrin monomer; monomers spontaneously polymerize by hydrogen bonding.

In the *intrinsic pathway*, coagulation may be initiated by the activation of Factor XII. In vitro, surface contact activates Factor XII. The activation process in vivo is not clear, but small amounts of Factor XII_a can activate prekallikrein (Fletcher factor) to form kallikrein, which further activates Factor XII. Then, Factor XI may be activated by Factor XII_a or by some other mechanism as yet undiscovered. (Factor XII is needed for intrinsic clotting in vitro but not in vivo; persons with Factor XII deficiency have no bleeding disorder. Therefore, an alternate path of activation must exist in vivo.) Factor XI_a activates Factor IX. A complex of Factor IX_a, Factor VIII, phospholipid, and calcium forms which converts Factor X to Factor X_a. The reaction sequence then continues as described above.

The fibrin polymer then is stabilized by Factor XIII_a, activated from Factor XIII by thrombin and calcium. Factor XIII_a catalyzes cross-linking peptide bond formation between adjacent fibrin monomers. Without Factor XIII, fibrin polymers may disassociate; they are soluble in 5 M urea or dilute acids. Patients lacking this factor have a serious bleeding disorder.

Tests of Clotting Factor Interaction

The bleeding time and the clotting time are not appropriate screening tests of plasma clotting factor interaction. The bleeding time measures the ability to form platelet plugs and is abnormal only if the quantity or function of the platelets is abnormal. The whole blood clotting time is prolonged only in instances of a severe deficiency of a plasma clotting factor and is not long in moderate deficiencies which are clinically significant.

In the *Quick prothrombin time test,* tissue thromboplastin and calcium are added to citrated patient plasma and the time of appearance of fibrin strands is noted. The *extrinsic* pathway of clotting is being tested. The patient's plasma supplies Factors VII, X, and V and prothrombin and fibrinogen.

In the *partial thromboplastin time test* (PTT), a phospholipid reagent (supplying the equivalent of platelet factor 3) and calcium are added to citrated patient plasma and the time of appearance of fibrin strands is noted. In an activated partial thromboplastin time, a surface-active powder such as kaolin is added to the mixture to ensure maximal activation of Factor XII. These tests measure the *intrinsic* pathway of clotting. The patient's plasma supplies Factors XII, XI, IX, VIII, X, and V and prothrombin and fibrinogen.

If the Quick prothrombin time test or the partial thromboplastin time test, or both, are abnormal, assays which are specific for the clotting factors implicated by these abnormalities are performed.

The *differential partial thromboplastin time* may be useful if the patient's PTT is decidedly prolonged and specific factor assays are not available immediately. The patient's plasma is mixed with an equal volume of plasma from a person who has a severe deficiency of Factor VIII but adequate amounts of Factors IX, XI, and XII. If the clotting time of this mixture is normal or nearly normal, the patient probably has a deficiency of Factor IX, XI, or XII, but an adequate amount of Factor VIII. The combined plasmas provide all necessary plasma clotting factors for this test. If the clotting time of the mixture is still decidedly prolonged, the test patient is probably deficient in Factor VIII. Similar tests may be performed using plasmas known to be deficient in Factor IX, XI, or XII. The use of serum or adsorbed plasma, as factor-deficient reagents, often leads to confusing results; naturally deficient plasma is preferable. The differential PTT technique is not appropriate if the patient has only slight prolongation of the PTT because results are likely to be confusing (Table 2-1).

Table 2-1. Differential PTT

	PTT
Patient John Doe	80 sec.
Normal plasma	40 sec.
Patient Doe and known Factor VIII deficient plasma	78 sec.
Patient Doe and known Factor IX deficient plasma	45 sec.

Conclusion: Patient Doe has factor VIII deficiency.

If the PTT is prolonged, a *screening test for inhibitor* should be performed. Most inhibitors can be detected by a modification of the PTT, as follows: An equal mixture of patient plasma and normal plasma is allowed to sit in a plastic tube at 37°C for an hour. Then, the PTT is measured and compared to the PTT of pure normal plasma which has been incubated similarly. If the patient has no inhibitor, the PTT of the mixture will be a few seconds longer than that of pure normal plasma. If the patient has an inhibitor, his plasma will destroy some of the Factor VIII (or Factor IX or other clotting factor or clotting intermediary) in the normal plasma mixture and the PTT of the mixture will be prolonged markedly (Table 2-2).

Table 2-2. Inhibitor tests

	PTT after 1 hr. at 37°C
Patient Smith	80 sec.
Patient Jones	80 sec.
Normal plasma	40 sec.
Patient Smith plus normal plasma	45 sec.
Patient Jones plus normal plasma	75 sec.

Conclusion: Patient Jones has an inhibitor.

A test for an inhibitor to a specific clotting factor may be performed by mixing patient plasma and normal plasma and assaying the clotting factor level in the mixture after incubation. For example, some clinically significant mild inhibitors of Factor VIII may be detected by the following technique: Four parts of patient plasma and one part of normal plasma are mixed in a plastic tube and the Factor VIII level is assayed. The mixture is allowed to incubate one hour at 37°C and the Factor VIII level is measured again; unless an inhibitor is present, no Factor VIII is lost. The mixture is then refrigerated at 4°C for 23 hours and the Factor VIII level is assayed again. Unless an inhibitor is present, the Factor VIII level should be at least half that present in the mixture at the beginning of the test. If the Factor VIII level is less than a quarter of that present at the beginning of the test, an inhibitor may be diagnosed (Table 2-3).

In the *thrombin time test*, dilute thrombin is added to citrated patient plasma and the time of appearance of fibrin strands is noted. The clotting time is prolonged if there is severe hypofibrinogenemia or qualitatively abnormal fibrinogen. The test is also sensitive to the presence of small amounts of heparin in the plasma and to the presence of fibrin split products (which interfere with the polymerization of fibrin monomer.)

A *fibrinogen titer* is a better way of estimating the fibrinogen level in plasma than the thrombin time, prothrombin time, or PTT. These screening tests may be normal when fibrinogen deficiency is moderately severe.

The adequacy of Factor XIII is tested by recalcifying citrated patient plasma and allowing a clot to form. The clot is then suspended in 5 M urea or in 1 percent monochloracetic acid; the clot should remain intact at room temperature for 24 hours. Deficiency of Factor XIII is *not* revealed by any of the other screening tests described above.

Table 2-3. Inhibitor assay

	Factor VIII		
	Zero time	1 hour	24 hours
1 part normal plasma plus 4 parts plasma patient Smith	20%	20%	10%
1 part normal plasma plus 4 parts plasma patient Jones	20%	17%	2%

Conclusion: Patient Jones has a mild inhibitor.

Tests of Platelet Function

A *platelet count* will determine whether there are enough platelets to carry out their functions in clotting. A *bleeding time* is a test of the ability of platelets to form a plug. The time may be prolonged if platelets are inherently defective or are too few in number, or if platelets have been affected by agents toxic to them, such as aspirin, or if the platelets lack a plasma substance necessary for their function, as in von Willebrand's disease.

In the *platelet adhesiveness test,* the platelet count of fresh venous blood is compared to that of blood which has been passed through a column of glass beads. Normally, the percentage of platelets adhering to the beads is high. In von Willebrand's disease, adherence is low. Platelets normally aggregate when exposed to such agents as adenosine diphosphate, collagen, epinephrine, ristocetin, and others. Aggregation with ristocetin usually is reduced in von Willebrand's disease whereas aggregation with other agents is normal. Patients with inherently defective platelets may have poor platelet adhesiveness, poor aggregation with one or several agents, abnormalities in tests for decreased storage of lipid, or inadequate release of lipid, or several of these defects.

DIAGNOSIS OF THE COMMON HEMOPHILIAS

Hemophilia A (Classic Hemophilia, Sex-Linked Factor VIII Deficiency)

In Hemophilia A, the patient's plasma is deficient in Factor VIII clotting activity but contains normal amounts of an antigen which precipitates with a rabbit antihuman Factor VIII antibody. This finding suggests that the patient makes a Factor VIII molecule which is unable to function normally in the coagulation process.

The degree of Factor VIII deficiency is similar in all affected males in a given kindred. In some families, the deficiency is severe, and affected males have frequent joint and tissue hemorrhages which can lead to crippling deformities. Small cuts usually do not bleed excessively. In other families, the deficiency is moderate or mild, and affected males may bleed only after trauma or at surgical operations. Normal persons have Factor VIII levels ranging from about 50 to about 200 percent. Patients with hemophilia have Factor VIII levels from a fraction of 1 percent to 30 percent of the average normal level.

Screening tests for hemostatic function in hemophilia reveal normal bleeding time, prothrombin time, and thrombin time but a prolonged partial thromboplastin time. An assay specific for Factor VIII should be performed to determine the level of deficiency. About 8 percent of patients with severe classic hemophilia develop antibodies to Factor VIII (inhibitors) which inactivate infused Factor VIII.

The disorder is transmitted as a sex-linked recessive trait on the X chromosome. The children of a hemophilic man (genotype X^hY) and a normal woman (XX) can be either males (XY) with the father's Y chromosome or females (X^hX) with the father's affected X chromosome. Thus, all the sons will be free of hemophilia and cannot transmit the disorder to their descendants. All daughters are obligatory carriers.

The children of a normal man ($X_{fa}Y_{fa}$) and a carrier woman ($X_{mo}^h X_{mo}$) have equal chances of being normal males ($X_{mo}Y_{fa}$) or hemophilic males ($X_{mo}^h Y_{fa}$) or normal females ($X_{mo}X_{fa}$) or carrier females ($X_{mo}^h X_{fa}$).

Most carriers have Factor VIII levels in the 30 to 70 percent range. Some have higher levels, and some have levels below 30 percent and bleed excessively with trauma or surgical operations. If a potential carrier, for example, the sister of a hemophiliac, is found to have a Factor VIII level below the normal range, she may be told she is definitely a carrier. If the level is in the normal range, she can be given a statistical estimate of the probability that she is a carrier. In some laboratories, a test for Factor VIII antigen, using the rabbit antibody mentioned above, is available. This test probably measures the sum of normal and abnormal Factor VIII molecules; we presume that most carriers make both normal and abnormal Factor VIII molecules and that the level of Factor VIII measured as antigen should be higher than the level measured as Factor VIII activity. (In normal women, who make only normal Factor VIII molecules, the antigen and activity levels should be the same). If the level of Factor VIII antigen is significantly higher than the Factor VIII activity in a potential carrier, she can be told she is probably a true carrier. There is no test which enables us to tell a woman she is definitely not a carrier.

Assays for carrier detection should be performed only by laboratories experienced in these procedures. Women should not be tested during pregnancy or the puerperium.

Hemophilia B (Christmas Disease, Factor IX or PTC Deficiency)

In Hemophilia B, the patient's plasma is deficient in Factor IX clotting activity. In affected males in some families, an abnormal molecule can be detected by immunologic techniques. In other families, no abnormal molecules have been detected.

The clinical findings, genetic pattern and laboratory screening test findings in hemophilia B are parallel to those in hemophilia A, with few exceptions: (1) only 1 or 2 percent of patients with hemophilia B develop inhibitors to Factor IX and (2) carriers can be detected by immunologic techniques only in families in which an abnormal molecule can be detected in affected males.

Factor XI Deficiency (Hemophilia C, PTA Deficiency)

In hemophilia C, the patient's plasma is deficient in Factor XI clotting activity. No abnormal Factor XI molecules have been described as yet. Patients with Factor XI deficiency have prolonged bleeding after trauma or surgical operation. Unprovoked bleeding into deep tissues is uncommon even in severe deficiency of Factor XI.

Inheritance is of the autosomal recessive pattern, affecting both males and females. Parents and children of the patient will be heterozygous with low-normal levels of Factor XI (e.g., 50 percent) of no clinical significance.

Characteristic laboratory findings include a normal bleeding time, normal platelet function tests, and a normal prothrombin time but a prolonged PTT. If a differential PTT is performed with plasmas from patients with known deficiencies of Factor VIII and of Factor IX, correction may be obtained with both plasmas, though they may not correct equally well. A specific Factor XI assay should be obtained whenever this disorder is suspected.

Factor XII Deficiency (Hageman Factor Deficiency)

Persons with this deficiency are discovered accidentally when a routine partial thromboplastin time or a whole blood clotting time is prolonged. There is no tendency to bleed excessively. Inheritance is autosomal and recessive.

Deficiencies of Other Single Clotting Factors

Other deficiencies of single plasma clotting factors are extremely rare and are usually autosomal recessive traits. In homozygous Factor VII deficiency, the prothrombin time is prolonged but the partial thromboplastin time is normal. These persons have a severe bleeding disorder, thus demonstrating that both the extrinsic pathway and the intrinsic pathway are needed for adequate hemostasis in vivo. Patients with severe deficiency of Factor X or Factor V or prothrombin will have prolongation of the partial thromboplastin time and especially of the prothrombin time. In severe fibrinogen deficiency, these tests and the thrombin time may be prolonged. Factor XIII deficiency causes excessive bleeding and poor wound healing. This defect is detected only by a specific screening test for Factor XIII and not by the prothrombin time, the partial thromboplastin time or the thrombin time.

Von Willebrand's disease

This disorder is characterized by poor platelet plug formation and a variable degree of Factor VIII deficiency. The disorder of platelet plug formation leads to excessive bleeding from small cuts and mucosal abrasions and to heavy menstrual bleeding in females. In patients with very low Factor VIII levels, bleeding into joints and muscles may occur. All patients risk excessive bleeding from surgical procedures, including tooth extraction.

The platelet dysfunction is demonstrated by a prolonged bleeding time, by decreased retention of platelets by glass bead columns (platelet adhesiveness), and by decreased platelet aggregation with ristocetin (although aggregation is normal with other reagents.) The abnormal adhesiveness and ristocetin aggregation can be corrected by suspending the patient's platelets in normal plasma. Although infusion of normal plasma stops most hemorrhages, the bleeding time may remain long.

If the Factor VIII level is below 30 percent, the partial thromboplastin time is likely to be prolonged; the prothrombin time and the thrombin time are normal. In contrast to classic hemophilia, the lack of Factor VIII activity is associated with a comparable lack of antigen reacting with rabbit antibody. This finding suggests that patients with von Willebrand's disease produce less than normal amounts of Factor VIII molecule, whereas patients with classic hemophilia produce normal amounts of an abnormal Factor VIII molecule. In von Willebrand's disease, transfusion with normal plasma results in increased synthesis of Factor VIII by the patient for one or more days. The plasma factor missing in von Willebrand's disease, that factor which corrects the platelet dysfunction and stimulates Factor VIII production, is closely related in some way to the normal Factor VIII molecule.

Von Willebrand's disease is inherited as an autosomal disorder, usually dominant in mild or moderately affected families, and recessive in the most severely affected patients. Males and females can be equally affected. In contrast to sex linked hemophilia, Factor VIII levels vary from one affected person to another within the same family. Factor VIII levels and bleeding times also vary from time to time in the same person. An afflicted person might have an abnormal bleeding time and subnormal Factor VIII level on one occasion, and, on another occasion, have test results within normal limits. Platelet adhesiveness usually remains abnormal on all occasions.

Differential Diagnosis

Rare hereditary plasma clotting factor deficiencies may be detected by abnormality of the Quick prothrombin test, the PTT, the fibrinogen level, or a specific screening test for fibrin stabilizing factor. Acquired plasma clotting factor deficiencies may occur due to inadequate production of clotting factors (liver failure), to autoantibodies to clotting factors (systemic lupus erythematosis), or to rapid consumption or lysis of clotting factors (disseminated intravascular coagulation).

Rare hereditary defects of platelet function are characterized by long bleeding times and abnormalities of one or more platelet function tests, but the prothrombin time and PTT are normal. Acquired platelet defects include thrombocytopenia as well as defects of platelet function, as may occur in uremia.

TREATMENT OF HEMORRHAGES

Hemophilia A (Factor VIII Deficiency)

Minor, superficial hemorrhages, such as small skin cuts, may respond to prolonged pressure and cool packs. More extensive or deep hemorrhages are treated by replacing the missing clotting factor. The sooner the bleeding is stopped, the less damage will be done to the tissues, so treatment should be given at the first indication of a hemorrhage. The symptoms of hemorrhage, such as pain and stiffness in a joint or muscle, are felt hours before any swelling can be seen; the physician should start treatment when the patient declares he is bleeding. Factor VIII must be given intravenously in the form of normal human plasma or plasma concentrate. A mild superficial or very early hemorrhage sometimes will subside if a Factor VIII level of around 15 to 20 percent is achieved, but the episode will more surely subside if a level of 30 percent or more is attained. For any serious hemorrhage, a Factor VIII level of 35 to 50 percent should be obtained to permit the formation of an optimal clot. One adequate dose of Factor VIII is sufficient to treat most hemorrhages. However, Factor VIII is rapidly metabolized in the body with a half-disappearance time from the plasma of about eight hours. If the patient bleeds again several hours after the initial dose, he may require another dose of Factor VIII to achieve a satisfactory level.

Minor operations, such as tooth extraction or removal of a nevus, can be permitted with a single dose of Factor VIII given immediately before the procedure. Another dose of Factor VIII is given only if bleeding occurs. Rebleeding is most common on postoperative days five, six, and seven; the patient should avoid stress on the site for 10 days.

For more *extensive operations,* the factor VIII level is maintained at a daily minimum of at least 30 percent for a healing period of 10 to 14 days; Factor VIII levels are checked by specific factor assay. The first dose of Factor VIII, to achieve a level of 80 to 100 percent, is given an hour before the procedure; the plasma Factor VIII level is checked by assay. A second dose of Factor VIII, half the size of the priming dose, should be given about five hours after the priming dose. The patient may be in the recovery room by this time, or still in the operating room. If several units of blood were lost during the operation, a third dose of concentrate should be given when the patient reaches the recovery room. A dose of concentrate is also given in the late evening. Concentrate administration is continued for 10 days for relatively minor procedures, such as Achilles tendoplasty, and for 14 days for more extensive procedures, such as oste-

otomy. Concentrate is usually administered every 12 hours in a sufficient dose to maintain a minimum plasma Factor VIII level of at least 30 percent. The patient's hematocrit may fall slowly for several days after the operation without obvious bleeding. The patient adjusts his total blood volume by adding to his plasma volume; this enlargement of the plasma volume must be considered in the calculation of postoperative concentrate dosage. Patients undergoing postoperative rehabilitation, namely physical therapy, receive daily concentrate throughout the period of rehabilitation. (Fig. 2-2).

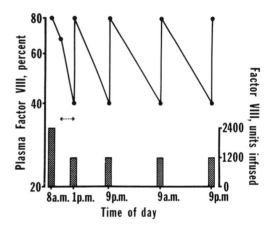

Figure 2-2. Schedule of Factor VIII administration and hypothetical plasma Factor VIII levels for major surgical operation in severe classic hemophilia. The dotted line indicates the period of time in the operating room. The solid lines represent expected plasma Factor VIII levels, presuming a 4 hour half-disappearance time of Factor VIII during the surgical procedure, an 8 hour half-disappearance time on the first day of concentrate administration (before and after the surgical procedure), and a 12 hour half-disappearance time after the first few doses of Factor VIII have been given.

Many hemorrhages can be prevented if the patient is "converted" from severe to moderate or mild status by the administration of small doses of Factor VIII every day. For example, if a patient is transfused to a Factor VIII level of 10 percent in the morning, he may retain 5 percent by late afternoon and 2 percent by bedtime; some protection is provided during the most active part of the day. Prophylaxis is particularly appropriate for patients undergoing physical therapy and for patients with very frequent hemorrhages (Fig. 2-3).

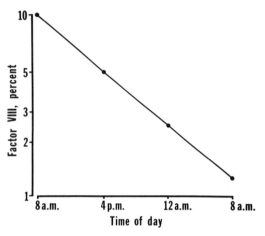

Figure 2-3. Hypothetical plasma Factor VIII levels, suitable for prophylaxis during the day, in a patient with severe classic hemophilia who was infused with sufficient Factor VIII to achieve a plasma level of 10 percent at 8 a.m.

Choice of Materials and Dosage

Three types of plasma products are available for the treatment of hemophilia A: fresh-frozen plasma, cryoprecipitate, and lyophilized Factor VIII concentrate.

Fresh-frozen plasma is obtained from blood banks. Each bag contains about 175 to 250 ml of plasma from one blood donation. The plasma should be stored at $-30°$ C. For administration to the patient, the bag of frozen plasma is placed in a pan of water at exactly 37°C. The bag, as it softens, may be manipulated to break up large chunks of frozen plasma in order to hasten thawing. Thawing should be complete since Factor VIII is among the last proteins to dissolve. The infusion of plasma should be prompt, because Factor VIII deteriorates at room temperature. The defrosted plasma may be expected to contain about 70 percent of the Factor VIII which was present in the fresh plasma. Different donors have different Factor VIII levels; the amount of Factor VIII in any given bag of frozen plasma is unpredictable.

Cryoprecipitate is prepared by blood banks. A bag of fresh plasma is quick fro-zen, then slowly thawed in a refrigerator until only a few milliliters of ice and sludge remain. This remaining material, or cryoprecipitate, contains about half the Factor VIII and fibrinogen which had been present in the fresh plasma. The thawed plasma is drained off; the cryoprecipitate is retained and refrozen. For administration to the patient, the bag is placed in a pan of water at exactly 37°C and allowed to thaw thoroughly (about 15 minutes). Sterile normal saline may be added to wash out bags containing a small volume of cryoprecipitate. The Factor VIII content of cryoprecipitate varies depending upon the donor's Factor VIII level and the blood bank's method of processing. With care, a blood bank should be able to produce cryoprecipitate averaging 100 AHF units per bag; however, this standard is often not attained.

Concentrates are prepared by the following pharmaceutical companies from pools of plasma obtained from a great many donors.

FACTOR VIII CONCENTRATES

Profilate—Abbott Scientific Products Division, 820 Mission Street, South Pasadena, California 91030 (213) 441-1171.

Factorate—Armour Pharmaceutical Company, Greyhound Tower, Phoenix, Arizona 85077 (602) 248-2820.

Koate—Cutter Laboratories, Inc., 4th and Parker Streets, Berkeley, California 94710 (415) 841-0123.

Hemofil—Hyland Division, Travenol Laboratories, Inc., Costa Mesa, California 92626 (714) 540-5000.

Humafac—Parke, Davis and Co., Detroit, Michigan 48232 (313) 567-5300.

Antihemophilic Factor (Human)—E. R. Squibb and Sons, Inc., New Brunswick, New Jersey, 08903 (609) 921-4066. Plasma collected by the American National Red Cross and distributed by the Red Cross Regional Blood Centers or from the National Headquarters, Washington, D.C. 20006 (202) 857-3348.

Factor VIII (with fibrinogen) is extracted and concentrated, distributed in 10 or 25 ml aliquots in glass vials, and lyophilized.

The vials are stored at refrigerator or room temperature. The concentrate is reconstituted with water or saline and administered intravenously. A sample bottle from each lot is assayed in vitro by the manufacturer, and the number of Factor VIII units is stamped on the label. (A Factor VIII, or AHF, unit is the amount of Factor VIII found in 1 ml of fresh average normal plasma.)

Several factors affect the choice of plasma product used to treat hemophilia A. The cardiovascular system cannot accept an unlimited volume of osmotically active fluid, such as plasma, at one time. If a 150 lb man with a 3000 ml plasma volume and a negligible Factor VIII level receives as much as 1000 ml of fresh-frozen plasma, containing 700 Factor VIII units, his resulting plasma Factor VIII level will be only 17.5 percent, whereas a higher level, over 30 percent, is desired to treat a serious hemorrhage. Patients with severe hemophilia are usually treated with cryoprecipitate and concentrate because a therapeutic level of Factor VIII can be achieved with a small volume of material. Patients with mild hemophilia, e.g., 20 percent Factor VIII, might be managed satisfactorily with plasma.

All blood products used in treating hemophilia can transmit the virus of serum hepatitis. Frozen plasma and cryoprecipitate are usually obtained from volunteer donors and not pooled prior to use; one infected donor can infect only one recipient. Concentrates are made from plasma pooled from a great many donors who are usually paid donors; one infected donor can infect all the recipients of the pool. Patients with severe hemophilia who require frequent infusions of plasma products will inevitably encounter the virus; they may as well receive concentrates. Patients with mild hemophilia who require treatment on few occasions should receive the single donor products.

Most hemophiliacs who have received many infusions of plasma develop allergic reactions such as hives and chills during infusions of plasma; they should be given antihistamines before infusion. Allergic reactions are infrequent with cryoprecipitate and rare with concentrate. Patients with blood types A, AB, or B should receive type-specific plasma to avoid hemolysis. Crossmatching is not indicated for plasma or cryoprecipitate.

Factor VIII content is not equally predictable in concentrate and cryoprecipitate. Concentrates can be relied upon to contain the approximate number of Factor VIII units stated on the label. Cryoprecipitate varies. The clinician should periodically assay the response of his patients to the cryoprecipitate available in his community to evaluate its potency.

Concentrate is more convenient for self-treatment because it can be transported at room temperature.

The price per Factor VIII unit varies among products and communities. The clinician faced with the high cost of treating severe hemophilia may want to seek the best bargain for his patient.

CALCULATION OF DOSAGE. To determine the number of Factor VIII units needed to achieve a desired plasma Factor VIII level, first estimate the patient's plasma volume, e.g., multiply weight in pounds times 20, and multiply by the percent Factor VIII increase desired. Examples:
Severe hemophiliac, negligible Factor VIII, 50 lbs:
   desire 30 percent Factor VIII level:
   $50 \times 20 \times 0.30 = 300$ AHF units needed.
Mild hemophiliac, 10 percent Factor VIII, 50 lbs:
   desires 30 percent Factor VIII level, i.e., increase from 10 percent to 30 percent:
   $50 \times 20 \times 0.20 = 200$ AHF units needed.

If a minimum level of Factor VIII is to be maintained over a prolonged period, estimate that the half-disappearance time of Factor VIII is 8 hours. With external blood loss or fever, the disappearance may be more rapid.

Severe hemophiliac, negligible Factor VIII, 50 lbs:
   desire maintenance of at least 30 percent Factor VIII:
   Initial dose, to achieve 60 percent

Table 2-4. Dosage calculation for concentrate or cryoprecipitate (Factor VIII units needed to raise plasma Factor VIII level to a desired level in lean male patients of various weights.)

Patient's weight (lbs)	Desired factor VIII level				
	20%	30%	40%	50%	60%
20	80 units	120 units	160 units	200 units	240 units
30	120	180	240	300	360
40	160	240	320	400	480
50	200	300	400	500	600
60	240	360	480	600	720
70	280	420	560	700	840
80	320	480	640	800	960
90	360	540	720	900	1080
100	400	600	800	1000	1200
110	440	660	880	1100	1320
120	480	720	960	1200	1440
130	520	780	1040	1300	1560
140	560	840	1120	1400	1680
150	600	900	1200	1500	1800
160	640	960	1280	1600	1920
170	680	1020	1360	1700	2040
180	720	1080	1440	1800	2160
190	760	1140	1520	1900	2280
200	800	1200	1600	2000	2400
220	880	1320	1760	2200	2640
240	960	1440	1920	2400	2800
260	1040	1560	2080	2600	3120

Factor VIII:
$50 \times 20 \times 0.60 = 600$ AHF units needed.
Next dose, eight hours later, to boost Factor VIII from 30 to 60 percent:
$50 \times 20 \times 0.30 = 300$ AHF units needed.
See Table 2-4.

Management of Inhibitors

Inhibitors are present in about 8 percent of patients with severe classic hemophilia. No one can predict who will develop an inhibitor, nor does anyone know how to prevent inhibitors. If a patient has the ability to develop a strong inhibitor, he probably will do so by the time he has been given plasma products on a hundred occasions or less. Since most patients with severe hemophilia in this country are treated vigorously for hemorrhages, this degree of exposure to plasma products usually will be achieved in early childhood. Severe inhibitors can appear in infants who have had only a few infusions; they can develop also in adults who have survived youth without extensive exposure to blood products. If a patient has received plasma products on at least a hundred occasions, and does not have an inhibitor, he probably will never develop a strong one. Weak inhibitors, on the other hand, may develop in older patients who have had hundreds of plasma infusions. Patients with inhibitors do not bleed more often than patients without them. An inhibitor state should be suspected when a patient fails to stop bleeding after an adequate infusion of plasma concentrate.

WEAK INHIBITORS IN HEAVILY TRANSFUSED PATIENTS. Those adolescent or adult patients who have received over a hundred infusions of plasma products and have been discovered to have a weak inhibitor may be able to receive further plasma products. Two philosophies exist about management of further plasma product infusions. According to one hypothesis, the patient should be given the same dose of Factor VIII as a patient of the same weight who does not have an inhibitor, that is, a "normal" dose. This Factor VIII will be inactivated by the patient's inhibitor within a few minutes. Therefore, an assay performed on the patient's plasma, drawn immediately after the infusion and rapidly processed, may detect no circulating Factor VIII. However, the Factor VIII may have participated in coagulation during its few minutes of survival. Other clinicians, dissatisfied with the effect of "normal" doses of Factor VIII, administer two or three times the normal dose to achieve a circulating Factor VIII level in the hemostatic range. Whichever policy is followed, the clinician should check the patient's inhibitor titer two weeks after the plasma product infusion. If the titer does not rise, the patient can continue to receive Factor VIII for the treatment of serious hemorrhages.

WEAK INHIBITORS IN SMALL CHILDREN OR MINIMALLY EXPOSED PATIENTS. If a weak inhibitor is detected in a small child, or in an older patient who has had very few infusions, one should presume that this early appearance indicates that the patient has a pronounced ability to form the antibody; he will probably develop a high titer inhibitor if he is given the opportunity by further exposure to Factor VIII. Minor hemorrhages can be managed with conservative measures and moderate doses of oral prednisone for a few days. For very serious hemorrhages, the patient may be given a normal dose, or a large dose of Factor VIII. An increase in inhibitor titer will probably occur in a few days. In most instances, cyclophosphamide has not been effective in preventing a rise in inhibitor titers; cyclophosphamide can cause serious side effects.

Reports from several hemophilia centers indicate that prothrombin complex concentrates (Factor IX concentrates used to treat hemophilia B) often stop hemorrhages in patients with hemophilia A and an inhibitor. Prothrombin complex concentrates contain activated clotting factors, probably including Factor X_a, which promote clotting at a stage in the interaction of clotting factors beyond the point of action of Factor VIII. Activated clotting factors probably circulate in the blood for only a few minutes before they are inactivated, but they may be able to stimulate clotting in the injured vessel within that short time. The dosage of Factor IX concentrate used to treat a hemorrhage in a patient with inhibitor is the same amount which would be given to a patient with hemophilia B of the same weight suffering a severe hemorrhage, that is, enough to raise the plasma Factor IX level from zero to 50 percent. If bleeding does not stop, the dose may be repeated, or a dose twice as large given. This use of prothrombin complex is still experimental. The side effects of prothrombin complex concentrate are described below. The titer of Factor VIII inhibitor usually does not rise after the use of Factor IX concentrate.

STRONG INHIBITORS. Patients with strong inhibitors do not benefit from Factor VIII infusions. The Factor VIII is rapidly destroyed in the circulation by the high titer antibody and probably has no chance to participate in coagulation. Prothrombin complex concentrate may promote hemostasis.

Hemophilia B (Factor IX Deficiency)

In principle, the management of hemophilia B is similar to that of hemophilia A. A Factor IX level of 30 percent is desirable for minor hemorrhages, and 50 percent for major ones. The disappearance pattern of Factor IX from the plasma differs from that of Factor VIII. Factor IX has a two-phase disappearance: an initial rapid disappearance with a half-life of about 4.5 hours, during which there is equilibration with extravascular spaces; and a second biologic disappearance with a half-life of about 32 hours. This complicated disappearance pattern need not trouble the clinician in determining dosages of Factor IX. The dosage and schedule of administration of Factor IX for acute hemorrhages or surgery is the same as that of Factor VIII in classic hemophilia. However, the slow biologic half-life of Factor IX is an advantage in prophylaxis; a once weekly dose of Factor IX prevents many hemorrhages in patients with severe hemophilia B.

Choice of Materials

There are two products available to treat hemophilia B: fresh-frozen plasma and lyophilized Factor IX concentrate (prothrombin complex concentrate).

Fresh plasma, the plasma remaining from preparation of cryoprecipitate, or plasma from "outdated" bank blood can be frozen and stored for use in hemophilia B. Factor IX is more stable than Factor VIII and survives well at refrigerator temperature. The method of administration of plasma and its advantages and disadvantages are the same as in classic hemophilia.

Concentrates containing Factor IX, as well as Factors II, VII, and X, are produced by pharmaceutical companies:

FACTOR IX CONCENTRATES (PROTHROMBIN COMPLEX CONCENTRATES)

Konyne—Cutter Laboratories, Inc., 4th and Parker Streets, Berkeley, California 94710 (415) 841-0123

Proplex—Hyland Division, Travenol Laboratories, Inc., Costa Mesa, California 92626 (714) 540-5000

Each lot of concentrate is produced from pooled plasma donations; aliquots are lyophilized in glass vials and assayed in vitro by the manufacturer. About one half of the Factor IX assayed in vitro is activated Factor IX, which is rapidly destroyed in the body and not detectable in the patient's plasma a few minutes after infusion. Therefore, the clinician must administer twice as much Factor IX, according to the in vitro assay, as he would have calculated in order to achieve a desired plasma Factor IX level.

FACTORS IN CHOICE OF MATERIAL. Plasma and concentrate have many of the same advantages and disadvantages as described in the treatment of hemophilia A. Patients with severe hemophilia B use concentrates in order to achieve satisfactory hemostatic levels of Factor IX. Patients with mild hemophilia, who rarely need transfusion, should be given single donor plasma, if possible, to minimize the risk of hepatitis. Factor IX concentrates require refrigeration.

We do not perform elective surgery on patients with severe hemophilia B because we have observed an increased incidence of postoperative venous thrombi and pulmonary emboli in patients receiving Factor IX concentrates. When a patient with hemophilia B required emergency surgery, we prepared him by infusing as much fresh-frozen plasma as his blood volume could tolerate and then infusing enough Factor IX concentrate to achieve a plasma Factor IX level of 50 percent. We added ten units of heparin to each 1 ml of reconstituted concentrate before infusion. In the postoperative period, we infused plasma every eight hours.

Factor IX concentrates may also induce venous thrombi or disseminated intravascular coagulation in patients with liver dysfunction. Many hemophiliacs have evidence of some degree of liver dysfunction as a result of past episodes of hepatitis. The International Society for Thrombosis and Haemostasis has recommended that ten units of heparin be added to each ml of reconstituted prothrombin complex before infusion. (Heparin should not be added if the concentrate is being used to treat a patient with a Factor VIII inhibitor.)

Factor XI (PTA) Deficiency

No concentrate containing Factor XI is available. Patients are treated with fresh-frozen plasma. A serious hemorrhage in a severely deficient patient should be treated with the maximum volume of plasma he can tolerate; for example, 1000 ml in a young man of 150 lbs. If the patient cannot tolerate a large infusion, and does not respond to a small one, his own deficient plasma can be exchanged for normal plasma by means of plasmapheresis.

Von Willebrand's Disease

The low Factor VIII level, the long bleeding time, and the low platelet adhesiveness in this disease are not equally easy to treat.

A low factor VIII level is easily corrected. An infusion of plasma, cryoprecipitate, or Factor VIII concentrate will result in the predicted rise in Factor VIII level and, within the next 24 hours, a secondary rise in Factor VIII, and then, within a few days, slow return to the patient's baseline level. The normal plasma or Factor VIII concentrate contains a substance which permits the manufacture of Factor VIII by the patient (Fig. 2-4).

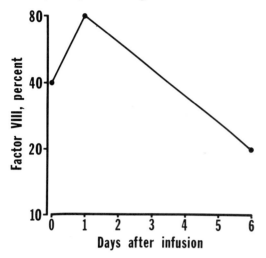

Figure 2-4. Plasma Factor VIII levels in a patient with severe von Willebrand's disease, who was transfused on day zero with an amount of cryoprecipitate calculated to raise his plasma Factor VIII level from less than 1 percent to 40 percent.

A low platelet adhesiveness will be improved by plasma or large doses of cryoprecipitate. Lyophilized concentrate is less effective. The platelets are not intrinsically defective; a factor present in normal plasma confers normal adhesiveness on platelets from patients with von Willebrand's disease. The maximum correction occurs about two or three hours after the infusion and the effect disappears within another couple of hours. The bleeding time may or may not respond to plasma, but if it improves, the duration of response is about the same as that of the platelet adhesiveness (Fig. 2-5).

For the treatment of *acute hemorrhages* in patients with a mild Factor VIII deficiency, fresh-frozen plasma may serve to correct the Factor VIII deficiency as well as the platelet dysfunction. Patients with severe Factor VIII deficiency may require cryoprecipitate to achieve an adequate immediate plasma level of Factor VIII. Bleeding from nose or mouth is especially

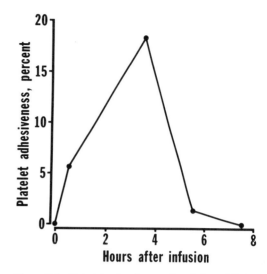

Figure 2-5. Platelet adhesiveness levels in a 50 lb boy with von Willebrand's disease after infusion of 225 ml of normal human plasma.

likely to recur in a few hours when the platelet adhesiveness returns to the low baseline, because platelet dysfunction is more significant than a mild Factor VIII deficit in mucosal hemorrhage. Patients with severe Factor VIII deficiency and musculoskeletal hemorrhages similar to those seen in severe hemophilia should be given a weekly infusion of plasma. The Factor VIII level will remain adequately elevated; Factor VIII is more significant than platelet function in prevention of musculoskeletal hemorrhage.

For surgery, the Factor VIII is maintained at a normal level. In patients with mild von Willebrand's disease, plasma should be given before the operation and repeated during a lengthy operation to correct the platelet adhesiveness in order to assure good clot formation at the surgical site. After a major operation or one notorious for postoperative bleeding (e.g., tonsillectomy), plasma can be given two or three times a day. Patients with severe von Willebrand's disease (very low Factor VIII levels) are prepared for surgery with cryoprecipitate and receive plasma in the postoperative period. Surgical healing is usually normal even if the prolonged bleeding time is not corrected by the infused plasma.

Women with *heavy menses* may be

given estrogen and progesterone in high dosage in order to raise the Factor VIII level. If that treatment is insufficient or contraindicated, the woman may be given epsilon-amino-caproic acid during menses. A dose of plasma at the onset of menses may be needed. A rare patient with very severe disease may require hysterectomy.

During *pregnancy,* the patient's Factor VIII level usually rises and may reach hemostatic levels. The bleeding time may or may not improve. If the bleeding time is still prolonged at term, the patient may need plasma for delivery.

Other Hereditary Bleeding Disorders

Deficiency of fibrinogen may be treated with cryoprecipitate, which is rich in fibrinogen. Deficiency of prothrombin or of Factor VII or of Factor X could be treated either with fresh-frozen plasma or with prothrombin complex concentrates, but the latter present the risks of serum hepatitis and thromboembolic disease. Deficiency of Factor V or Factor XIII can be treated with fresh-frozen plasma.

Patients with intrinsic platelet defects require transfusions of normal platelets to achieve hemostasis. The donor's blood and tissue types should be matched carefully to those of the recipient to prevent the development of platelet antibodies in the patient.

Oral Medications in Bleeding Disorders

Prednisone is given orally to reduce inflammation produced by a hemorrhage. An intravenous dose of a corticosteroid may be used to rapidly reduce swelling around a hemorrhage if the hemorrhage is compressing a vital structure, such as the trachea.

Epsilon-amino-caproic acid (EACA) inhibits the activation of plasminogen to plasmin, the body's natural fibrinolytic agent. A clot will remain intact longer if EACA is present. EACA does not assist in the formation of a clot. EACA should not be used if clotting occurs in an area where eventual resorption of the clot is desirable, e.g. the renal tubules. EACA is useful for patients having tooth extractions or in small children with a bleeding tongue or a lacerated frenulum. A dose of 40 mg/kg/day, up to a maximum of 10 gm/day given as an oral suspension, suffices for these purposes.

High-dosage estrogen-progesterone drugs may be useful in female patients to raise the level of Factor VIII or IX.

Some patients take aspirin or indomethacin to reduce the pain or stiffness of hemophilic arthritis. Both drugs prolong the bleeding time by interfering with platelet function. In severe hemophiliacs, the bleeding time may be extremely prolonged after a small dose of aspirin and remain long for two or three days. Acetaminophen, propoxyphene, and codeine do not affect the bleeding time and may be used for pain relief in hemophilia. Many patients feel that the relief from arthritic symptoms afforded by indomethacin outweighs the possible increase in bleeding tendency due to platelet dysfunction.

BIBLIOGRAPHY

Abildgaard, Charles F., Simone, Joseph V., Corrigan, James J., Seeler, Ruth A., Edelstein, Gerald, Vanderheiden, Jane, and Schulman, Irving: Treatment of hemophilia with glycine-precipitated Factor VIII. N. Engl. J. Med. 275:471, 1966.

Aggeler, Paul M.: Physiologic basis for transfusion therapy in hemorrhagic disorders: A critical review. Transfusion 1:71, 1961.

Aggeler, Paul M., Hoag, M. Silvija, Wallerstien, Ralph O., and Whissell, Dorothy: The mild hemophilias. Occult deficiencies of AHF, PTC and PTA frequently responsible for unexpected surgical bleeding. Am. J. Med. 30:84, 1961.

Barrow, Emily M., and Graham, John B.: Blood coagulation Factor VIII (antihemophilic factor): with comments on von Willebrand's disease and Christmas disease. Physiol. Rev. 54:23, 1974.

Blatt, Philip M., Lundblad, Roger L., Kingdon, Henry S., McLean, George, and Roberts, Harold R.: Thrombogenic materials in prothrombin complex concentrates. Ann. Intern. Med. 81:766, 1974.

Brown, Paul E., Hougie, Cecil, and Roberts, Harold R.: The genetic heterogeneity of hemophilia B. N. Engl. J. Med. 283:61, 1970.

Colman, Robert W.: Immunologic heterogeneity of hemophilia. N. Engl. J. Med. 288:369, 1973.

Croom, Robert D., III, and Hutchin, Peter: Surgical

management of the patient with classical hemophilia. Surg. Gynecol. Obstet. 128:793, 1969.

Dallman, Peter R., and Pool, Judith Graham: Treatment of hemophilia with Factor VIII concentrates. N. Engl. J. Med. 278:199, 1968.

Feinstein, Donald I., and Rapaport, Samuel I.: Acquired inhibitors of blood coagulation, in Spaet, T. H. (ed.): *Progress in Hemostasis and Thrombosis.* Grune & Stratton, New York, 1972.

Grammens, Gary R., and Breckenridge, Robert T.: Complications with Christmas factor (Factor IX) concentrates. Ann. Intern. Med. 80:666, 1974.

Hoag, M. Silvija, Johnson, Frederick F., Robinson, Jean A., and Aggeler, Paul M.: Treatment of hemophilia B with a new clotting factor concentrate. N. Engl. J. Med. 280:581, 1969.

Kaneshiro, M. M., Mielke, C. H., Jr., Kasper, C. K., and Rapaport, S. I.: Bleeding time after aspirin in disorders of intrinsic clotting. N. Engl. J. Med. 281:1039, 1969.

Kasper, Carol K.: Incidence and course of inhibitors among patients with classic hemophilia. Thromb. Diath. Haemorrh. 30:263, 1973.

Kasper, Carol K.: Postoperative thromboses in hemophilia B. N. Engl. J. Med. 289:160, 1973.

Kurczynski, Elizabeth M., and Penner, John A.: Activated prothrombin concentrate for patients with Factor VIII inhibitors. N. Engl. J. Med. 291:164, 1974.

Larrieu, M. J., Caen, J. P., Meyer, D. O., Vainer, H., Sultan, Y., and Bernard, Jean: Congenital bleeding disorders with long bleeding time and normal platelet count. II. Von Willebrand's disease (report of thirty-seven patients). Am. J. Med. 45:354, 1968.

Levine, Peter H., and Britten, Anthony F. H.: Supervised patient-management of hemophilia. A study of 45 patients with hemophilia A and B. Ann. Intern. Med. 78:195, 1973.

Meyer, Dominique, and Larrieu, Marie-José: Von Willebrand's factor and platelet adhesiveness. J. Clin. Pathol. 23:228, 1970.

Meyer, Dominique, Larrieu, Marie-José, Maroteaux, Pierre, and Caen, Jacques P.: Biological findings in von Willebrand's pedigrees: Implications for inheritance. J. Clin. Pathol. 20:90, 1967.

Perkins, Herbert A.: Correction of the hemostatic defects in von Willebrand's disease. Blood 30:375, 1967.

Pool, Judith Graham, and Shannon, Angela E.: Production of high-potency concentrates of anti-hemophilic globulin in a closed-bag system. Assay in vitro and in vivo. N. Engl. J. Med.

273:1443, 1965.

Rapaport, Samuel I., Patch, Mary Jane, and Moore, Frederick J.: Anti-hemophilic globulin levels in carriers of hemophilia A. J. Clin. Invest. 39:1619, 1960.

Rapaport, Samuel I., Proctor, Robert R., Patch, Mary Jane, and Yettra, Maurice: The mode of inheritance of PTA deficiency: Evidence for the existence of major PTA deficiency and minor PTA deficiency. Blood 18:149, 1961.

Ratnoff, Oscar D.: Hemophilia and von Willebrand's disease. West. J. Med. 120:226, 1974.

Rosenthal, Robert R., and Sloan, Esther: PTA (Factor XI) levels and coagulation studies after plasma infusions in PTA-deficient patients. J. Lab. Clin. Med. 66:709, 1965.

Schulman, Irving: Pediatric aspects of the mild hemophilias. Med. Clin. N. Am. 46:93, 1962.

Shulman, N. Raphael: The physiologic basis for therapy of classic hemophilia (Factor VIII deficiency) and related disorders. Ann. Intern. Med. 67:856, 1967.

Strauss, Herbert J.: The perpetuation of hemophilia by mutation. Pediatrics 39:186, 1967.

Strauss, Herbert S.: Acquired circulating anticoagulants in hemophilia A. N. Engl. J. Med. 281:866, 1969.

Strauss, Herbert S., and Bloom, Gerald E.: Von Willebrand's disease. Use of a platelet-adhesiveness test in diagnosis and family investigation. N. Engl. J. Med. 273:171, 1965.

Veltkamp, J. J., Drion, E. F., and Loeliger, E. A.: Detection of the carrier state in hereditary coagulation disorders. Thromb. Diath. Haemorrh. 19:279, 1968.

Walker, E. Helen, and Dormandy, Katharine M.: The management of pregnancy in von Willebrand's disease. J. Obstet. Gynecol. Br. Commonw. 75:459, 1968.

Weiss, Harvey J.: Abnormalities of Factor VIII and platelet aggregation-use of ristocetin in diagnosing the von Willebrand syndrome. Blood 45:403, 1975.

Zimmermann, Theodore S., Ratnoff, Oscar D., and Littell, Arthur S.: Detection of carriers of classic hemophilia using an immunologic assay for antihemophilic factor (Factor VIII). J. Clin. Invest. 50:255, 1971.

Zimmerman, Theodore S., Ratnoff, Oscar D., and Powell, Arnold E.: Immunologic differentiation of classic hemophilia (Factor VIII deficiency) and von Willebrand's disease. J. Clin. Invest. 50:244, 1971.

3

MEDICAL MANAGEMENT OF HEMOPHILIA

Shelby L. Dietrich

GENERAL PRINCIPLES

Hemophilic patients of all ages require regular medical supervision throughout their lives with attention focused on problems specific to the patient's age. Medical care *should not* be limited to sporadic, episodic emergency treatment of bleeding episodes; a schedule of regular annual or semiannual medical examinations should be maintained. The physician should keep in mind that his hemophilic patient is subject to the same diseases which afflict the general population. A close relationship between the physician and his patient is essential.

General guidelines for medical supervision of hemophilic patients include tests and procedures (e.g., immunizations, chest X-rays, etc.) appropriate for the patient's age, but one must also consider special problems inherent with hemophilia or related to the risks of treatment. All hemophilic patients have periodic tests of liver function, and special care is devoted to the abdominal examination to detect a palpable or enlarged liver or spleen. The presence of unsuspected iron deficiency, with or without anemia, may be confirmed by serum iron, iron-binding, and saturation tests. Those hemophilic patients who have frequent, small epistaxes or other bleeding episodes with external loss of blood are prone to this problem.

When the patient presents with an acute major bleeding episode, several sequential laboratory determinations of hemoglobin and hematocrit are useful aids in determining the volume of blood loss. A moderate degree of leukocytosis with "left shift" often is found with deep or large muscular hemorrhages or iliopsoas hemorrhages and does not necessarily denote infection.

MANAGEMENT OF HEMORRHAGE

Medical management of hemorrhage depends upon the following factors: (1) the diagnosis of the specific type and severity of the coagulation disorder, i.e., Factor VIII deficiency with an assayed VIII level less than 1 percent; (2) the presence or absence of an inhibitor to Factor VIII or IX; (3) the age and general health status of the patient including the presence of diseases not related to hemophilia. A careful history is obtained including evidence of trauma. The particular bleeding problem is evaluated keeping in mind such factors as: the site of hemorrhage, actual and potential blood volume loss, immediate problems, and long range sequelae.

The physical examination of the patient, including determination of pulse and respiratory rates and blood pressure, must include not only a general examination but, additionally, must focus on the area of suspected bleeding. It is helpful to remember that the patient's chief complaint or most obvious problem may not be the *only* site of hemorrhage as the following case history demonstrates:

A seven-year-old boy with severe Factor IX deficiency sustained an extensive linear skull fracture when he fell from a barn roof. He was hospitalized and observed closely because of signs of cerebral concussion (drowsiness, vomiting, and irritability) and treated with Factor IX concentrate. Six days after his accident, when he attempted to resume ambulation, he was noted to have a hip flexion contracture on the left side, displayed tenderness in the left lower abdominal quadrant, and evidenced a left thigh larger in size than the right one. Radiographs of the involved area revealed no fracture, so it was concluded that the patient had also suffered retroperitoneal and soft tissue hematomata at the time of his accident, which were undetected until the patient attempted to walk.

Visual inspection and comparison as well as manual palpation of joints and soft tissues will aid in detection of deep hemorrhages. Radiographs are helpful in differential diagnosis in many instances. A flat plate of the abdomen may outline the margins of the iliopsoas muscles and thereby aid in the diagnosis of iliopsoas (or retroperitoneal) hemorrhage. An anteroposterior view of the pelvis will include both hip joints and enable one to compare the joint spaces, the acetabula, and the femoral heads. At all times, radiologic interpretation should be correlated with the clinical history and examination.

Concentrate dosages are calculated for minor and major bleeding episodes according to body weight and estimated plasma volume. Factor levels of 30 percent are usually adequate for minor bleeding problems which include all hemarthroses except the hip, the soft tissue areas of the extremities, and external oropharyngeal bleeding. A dosage of concentrate to attain factor levels of 50 percent of normal is necessary for major hemorrhagic problems including cranial, submucosal oropharyngeal, intestinal, iliopsoas, retroperitoneal, kidney, and deep muscle areas; repeated infusions may be required depending upon the location, severity, and resolution of the hemorrhage. Detailed management of minor bleeding episodes is covered in Chapter 4, Nursing Care; however, certain major problems deserve special note.

A rare but potentially serious complication of hemophilia is the occurrence of *hemophilic pseudotumors* or *hemophilic cysts*. Management of these tumors as well as a review of the cases at this Center can be found in Chapter 8.

Intracranial hemorrhage is the leading cause of hemophilic mortality at the Orthopaedic Hospital. The onset of bleeding may be causally related to trauma, but in many instances no causal relationship can be established. With any indication of cerebral trauma or unusual cerebral symptoms, intracranial bleeding is suspected and the patient is treated vigorously. He is usually hospitalized; vital signs including blood pressure, respiratory and pulse rates, pupil size and reactivity, and the level of consciousness are checked and recorded at frequent intervals. Appropriate plasma products are infused to elevate the patient's factor level to 50 percent minimally. If localizing neurologic signs develop, surgical exploration and craniotomy for a possible subdural or epidural hematoma are performed. Electroencephalograms radioisotope brain scans, echoencephalograms, computerized arial tomograms, and occasionally carotid arteriograms, may help define the nature of the lesion. The following case illustrates management of this type of hemorrhage:

An 11-year-old boy with known severe hemophilia B was admitted to the hospital with a history of vomiting and severe headaches for the previous four days. There was no definite history of prior trauma although the patient remembered a mild blow to the head occurring at school. He was found to have aphasia and right-sided facial weakness. Immediate craniotomy with bilateral burr holes was performed following preparation with Factor IX concentrate. A subdural hematoma overlying the left hemisphere was evacuated. His subsequent hospital course was unremarkable except for one convulsive episode. The patient ultimately recovered completely from this intracranial lesion; no further convulsions have occurred in a three and a half year follow up.

Plasma products and other treatment are administered on the basis of head trauma and are not withheld until abnormal neurologic signs appear.

Other life-threatening hemorrhages relate to bleeding in and around the vital structures of the neck producing tracheal compression. Patients with respiratory embarrassment or difficulty in swallowing are admitted to the hospital; maximum therapy is instituted (Fig. 3-1). Intravenous administration of adrenocortical steroids (intravenous dexamethosone in an initial dose of 4 mg followed by 2 to 4 mg every 4 hours as indicated) may reduce pharyngeal or laryngeal edema. Antibi-

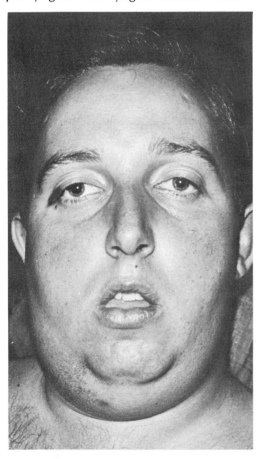

Figure 3-1. Adult with large submandibular and sublingual hematoma; "bull-neck" appearance and inability to close mouth are characteristic.

otics are administered if an infection is present. Plasma concentrates are infused every 12 hours until the dangers of respiratory complications are eliminated. A liquid diet is advised for 24 hours following the bleeding episode; next, cool, pureed foods are consumed until the hematoma has resolved.

Symptoms of *gastrointestinal* bleeding may include nausea, vomiting of dark red blood or "coffee-ground" like material, abdominal pain, or black, tarry stools. Severe blood loss or marked symptomatology always necessitates hospital admission. Plasma products are given every 12 hours until hemorrhage has resolved. Blood transfusions may be required. Extensive diagnostic tests are advised with recurrent gastrointestinal hemorrhage.

USE OF MEDICATIONS

Complaints of pain are evaluated and appropriate analgesia in adequate amounts is given. Aspirin or any compound containing salicylate is avoided because of its effect on platelet function. Patients are counseled to avoid common "over-the-counter" remedies, i.e., Anacin, Excedrin, "cold remedies," and Alka-Seltzer, since these contain aspirin.

Recommended medications for mild pain are acetaminophen or propoxyphene; for moderate to severe pain, codeine, pentazocine, meperidine, or morphine sulfate. Orally administered Dilaudid is also useful. Propoxyphene is not used in patients who are prone to drug abuse.

To reduce drug abuse and/or dependence, one physician assumes responsibility for the individual patient's analgesic prescriptions. Complete medication records are maintained in the outpatient treatment area. Whenever possible, the mildest analgesic is used. Except at times when the patient is hospitalized and under close medical supervision, excessive use of tranquilizers and barbiturates is discouraged. The genuine pain of an acute hemarthrosis or postoperative pain is relieved promptly with effective dosages of analgesics; greater than normal amounts of analgesic drugs may be required for adequate pain relief. Those patients who ingest codeine containing compounds on a daily basis in amounts totaling 200 to 300 mg may require morphine in 10 to 16 mg dosages or meperidine in a range of 100 to 150 mg every three hours for relief.

A realistic attitude toward pain should be developed by the patient with a chronic, painful disease, i.e., not all his chronic discomfort can be alleviated.

The physician must avoid assuming a punitive or judgmental attitude toward the patient who demands seemingly excessive amounts of analgesics. By setting firm limits and relieving acute severe pain promptly, both the physician and patient can develop attitudes of respect and confidence toward each other.

CARE OF THE PEDIATRIC HEMOPHILIAC

Infancy and Early Childhood to Age Five

Well-Child Care

Well-child care includes complete immunizations: diphtheria, tetanus, pertussis, poliomyelitis, mumps, measles, and rubella. Combined vaccines are used when possible, i.e., the diphtheria-pertussis-tetanus (DPT) series, the measles-mumps-rubella (M-M-R) series, and the tuberculin skin test. It is unnecessary to administer concentrate before immunizations because of the small volume of material injected. Intramuscular hematomas from vaccine injections are extremely rare. Parents are counseled regarding the usual febrile reaction to certain immunizations because an unusually severe local reaction to intramuscular vaccines, particularly DPT or tetanus toxoid, may be confused with a hematoma.

A dietary related iron deficiency coupled with frequent, small hemorrhages may predispose the child to iron deficiency anemia which is treated orally with ferrous sulfate, or other ferrous compounds, at a dosage of 5 mg per kg daily. Dietary counseling with the mother will help to prevent iron deficiency anemia by stressing the intake of adequate amounts of meat, eggs, and iron fortified cereals. Prolonged bottle feeding is discouraged.

Erupting or exfoliating deciduous teeth rarely cause gingival bleeding. Vigorous chewing will aid the eruption. Loose, exfoliating teeth which are causing bleeding should be extracted as discussed in Chapter 9, General Dental Care. Plasma concentrate is rarely indicated for these extractions.

Infections of Childhood

The hemophilic child is subject to the same diseases of childhood as any other child. Most mild respiratory or gastrointestinal infections are managed at home as are those of nonhemophilic children using appropriate dietary restrictions, cooling measures, and acetaminophen, instead of aspirin, to reduce temperature elevation. Concentrate or cryoprecipitate is seldom needed in the presence of an uncomplicated infection, but it is important to remember that some infections may predispose to bleeding and, conversely, some bleeding episodes may predispose to infection. The child with an intensely hyperemic pharynx, or greatly enlarged and injected tonsils, or injected tympanic membranes may hemorrhage into

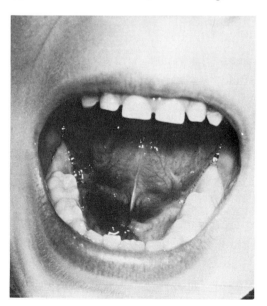

Figure 3-2. Child with small sublingual hemorrhage.

the sublingual, pharyngeal, or the sub-mandibular areas; swelling in the neck can be easily mistaken for "mumps" or epidemic parotitis (Fig. 3-2). An accurate diagnosis is essential for successful management of the problems.

Prolonged and severe coughing may precipitate hemorrhage into the throat or neck. Children with these conditions, combined with a greatly elevated temperature, toxicity, or dehydration are hospitalized and treated with intravenous penicillin or an acceptable alternative, and plasma concentrate. Infants and children with severe vomiting or diarrhea may also incur hemorrhage in the gastrointestinal tract; they are treated with hospitalization, concentrate, and intravenous fluids.

The common infectious diseases of childhood are either prevented by appropriate vaccine administration or may occur in a mild form in hemophilic children. Ordinarily, varicella, or chickenpox, produces mild symptoms, however, hand restraints may be necessary to prevent traumatic excoriation of lesions caused by scratching. Medications which control pruritus such as trimeprazine (Temaril) or diphenhydramine (Benadryl) may provide relief. Rubeola (measles) with severe enanthema may cause gastrointestinal bleeding which is managed by concentrate administration; however, measles can be adequately prevented by vaccine administration. Streptococcal infections of the tonsils or oropharynx may precipitate sublingual or oropharyngeal bleeding. Throat cultures are performed on all suspicious cases and oral penicillin, or an acceptable alternative, is administered even before the culture results are available. If bleeding is suspected or detected, concentrate is administered.

When the history and the physical examination suggest meningitis, the coagulation deficiency must be corrected before performing an atraumatic lumbar spinal tap. Factor levels of 50 percent are attained. Proven or suspected bacterial meningitis is managed in the customary manner. Occasionally, head injury with intracranial bleeding may simulate in-creased intracranial pressure from meningitis or encephalitis. Examination of the spinal fluid with appropriate gram stain and culture should differentiate these two entities. Until the diagnosis is clear, the patient is treated for both problems, i.e., administration of concentrate as well as appropriate intravenous antibiotics.

Convulsions may occur in hemophilic children from head trauma with intracranial bleeding, from febrile states, or as idiopathic seizures. Medication is chosen according to the nature and course of the seizures and continued until the patient has been seizure free for two or three years.

Management of Common Bleeding Problems

Circumcision in the neonatal period is avoided if a family history of hemophilia

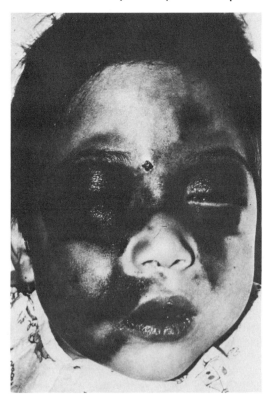

Figure 3-3. Extensive subcutaneous facial hemorrhage originating from a small laceration and contusion at the base of the nose.

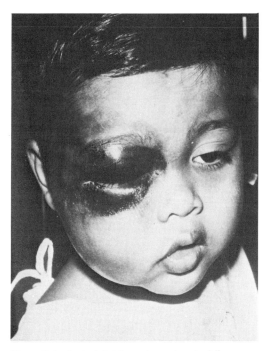

Figure 3-4. Periorbital hematoma in a toddler.

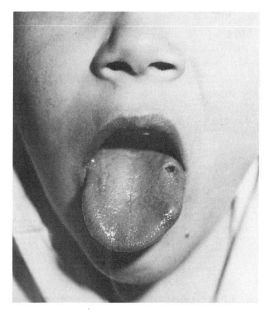

Figure 3-5. Laceration on the dorsum of the tongue which oozed persistently.

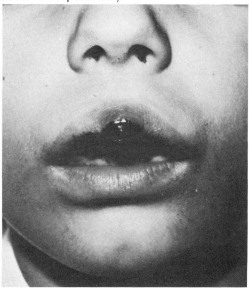

Figure 3-6. Laceration and contusion of the frenulum.

exists. If circumcision is inadvertently performed and produces continued bleeding, the correct diagnosis is established but the infant is treated on the basis of the family history by administration of either cryoprecipitate or fresh frozen plasma. Plasma concentrate preparations are avoided if at all possible in early infancy because of the danger of hepatitis and the baby's immature immunologic state.

Superficial lacerations of the face, mouth, tongue, or frenulum are annoying but generally minor problems of infancy and early childhood. (Figs. 3-3, 3-4, 3-5, and 3-6). These minor lacerations are treated every 12 hours for two or three doses of appropriate concentrate to levels of 30 to 50 percent, or every 24 hours with a larger dose to attain a level of approximately 100 percent. Generally, two or three days of this treatment is sufficient for healing. Minor lacerations of the tongue or oral mucosa are *not sutured* or cauterized. Local pressure may be helpful using topical thrombin preparations or oxidized, regenerated cellulose gauze (Surgicel). Large, raspberry-like, friable clots are removed manually from the tongue or mouth. Epsilon-amino-caproic acid is useful for management of these minor lacerations. A dosage of 38 mg/kg/day, up to a maximum of 10 gm/day, given as an oral suspension, suffices for these purposes. The child's hemoglobin and hematocrit are determined every 24 to 48 hours when bleeding persists from the mouth or lip. Since an infant's total blood volume is small, minor hemorrhages may lead to hemodilution and eventually hypovolemia. When whole blood transfusion is indicated, freshly packed red cells are preferred rather than whole blood in order to avoid transfusing unnecessary plasma elements and excess fluid volume. Restraints may be necessary to keep the child's hands from his mouth; chloral hydrate or promethazine suppositories are useful when sedation is required.

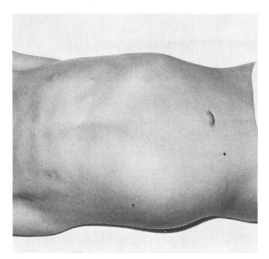

Figure 3-7. Asymmetry of abdominal wall characterizing intramuscular hematoma; costal margin on the right is not as well-defined as on the left side.

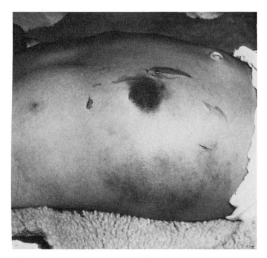

Figure 3-8. Massive intra-abdominal and intramuscular hematoma with subcutaneous discoloration; umbilicus shows early McEwen's sign (protrusion).

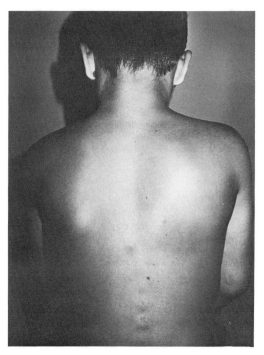

Figure 3-9. Right side periscapular hematoma.

Soft tissue hemorrhages of the thorax, the trunk, or the extremities may become extensive with minimal external evidence of such bleeding. Hemoglobin and hematocrit levels are watched carefully as are the child's general appearance, activity level, and presence or absence of pallor. Asymmetry of the body as well as general pallor often signal the presence of a large thoracic or abdominal hematoma (Figs. 3-7, 3-8, and 3-9).

If the history or the physical examination indicates the possibility of cerebral contusion or concussion, the child should be treated immediately with plasma concentrate and hospitalized for observation. Treatment should not be delayed until abnormal neurologic signs appear. Rarely, intracranial hemorrhage may occur secondary to birth trauma. Cephalohematoma in the newborn may result from the trauma of birth in a hemophilic infant. The pregnant mother with a family history of hemophilia should be advised to inform her obstetrician and her pediatrician of the possibility of a hemophilic infant so that circumcision will be avoided and other problems can be treated. When intracranial hemorrhage or large cephalohematoma occurs, cryoprecipitate or fresh frozen plasma are administered. The duration and frequency of such treatment will vary with the individual patient.

A rare but potentially extremely serious condition is epidural hemorrhage of the spinal cord precipitated by falling on the buttocks or falling into a sitting position with subsequent bleeding in the venous plexus of the epidural space of the spinal cord. Such hemorrhage may begin insidiously and the history of a fall as described may be difficult to elicit. If a patient with known hemophilia, especially in the toddler age, presents with either a history of a fall or with physical signs of soft tissue hematoma in the buttocks, careful attention should be paid to motor and sensory examination of the lower extremities. Follow-up examinations to determine any change in motor or sensory status of the lower extremities or involvement of bladder or bowel function are essential. If signs and symptoms of spinal cord or nerve root compression should appear, consideration should be given early to diagnostic myelogram with neurosurgical consultation and possible laminectomy. It must be emphasized that early awareness and suspicion of such a possibility will lead to early diagnosis and early intervention. Late intervention may well establish the diagnosis of spinal cord epidural hemorrhage but will do little to change the status of spinal cord function.

Middle Childhood, Ages 5 to 12

Well-child and preventive health care continue for the hemophilic as for any other child. The frequency and the type of examinations and immunizations are completely outlined in "Standards of Child Health Care" published by the American Academy of Pediatrics. In general, children of this age are healthy except for the occurrence of minor respiratory and gastrointestinal illnesses. When a child enters school at age four or five, he is immediately exposed and sus-

ceptible to many infecting organisms, chiefly viruses, with which he has had no previous contact. Therefore, one can expect an increased incidence of viral illness; parents may be reassured that such illness is not uncommon. If immunizations are complete and according to the schedule advised in "Standards of Child Health Care," chickenpox, streptococcal, and viral infections are the only common diseases against which the child has not developed immunity.

Tonsils and adenoids reach their maximum size during this age of childhood. Tonsillectomy and adenoidectomy, or adenoidectomy alone, are considered major undertakings in the child with hemophilia since the surgery will necessitate hospitalization and treatment with concentrate or cryoprecipitate for at least two weeks. Conservative treatment is vigorously pursued anticipating that the tonsils and adenoids will undergo natural regression and involution as the child grows older.

Bleeding Problems

An increased incidence of hemarthroses, particularly into knees and ankles, and of soft tissue hemorrhages of the extremities are found as the child increases his activities. Regular assessment of his musculoskeletal status assumes increasing importance. Intracranial hemorrhages may rarely appear without apparent antecedent cause and should be treated as previously described.

Genitourinary bleeding may appear; the episodes of hematuria may be frequent or prolonged. Treatment includes plasma concentrate administration and adequate fluid intake; a short course of prednisone may be helpful. Antifibrinolytic agents such as epsilon-amino-caproic acid are not used because of the possibility of clot formation in the ureter with subsequent renal or ureteral obstruction. Antimicrobial sensitivity tests are performed on urine cultures; renal function is evaluated by creatinine and blood urea nitrogen determinations. Intravenous pyelography is necessary with frequent recurrences or when clinical signs and symptoms for adequate diagnosis indicate as demonstrated by the following history:

A 13-year-old boy with severe Factor IX deficiency was admitted to the hospital with a seven day history of lower abdominal pain and urinary discomfort following voiding. Although there was no history of trauma or a fall, careful questioning of the patient revealed that prior to the onset of the present complaint, he had been riding a motorcycle. On admission, he had a temperature of 102° F and superpubic abdominal tenderness. Intravenous pyelogram revealed a "teardrop" shaped bladder consistent with pelvic hematoma. The patient was treated conservatively with Factor IX concentrate and rest; he improved rapidly during the five days of hospitalization. It is interesting that he presented no evidence of superficial hematoma formation in either the scrotum or the perineal region.

A problem of childhood which is almost unique to hemophilic boys is the occurrence of trauma induced hemorrhages of the scrotum from bicycle or tricycle riding. Occasionally, these hemorrhages may also occur following a straddle type injury. The patient's pain is promptly relieved, a scrotal suspensory or support is applied, and concentrate is administered on a daily basis until the hemorrhage appears to be resolving. Despite the massive appearing nature of these hemorrhages, permanent sequelae are extremely rare; no cases of testicular torsion or gangrene have been encountered in a hemophiliac at Orthopaedic Hospital as a result of this traumatic injury (Fig. 10A-C).

Major skin lacerations should be treated with concentrate administration for five to seven days in addition to suturing. When concentrate is not administered, a minor problem can turn into a major one because of the formation of a hematoma which interferes with primary wound healing.

Problems of the Adolescent Hemophiliac

Adolescent hemophilic boys have

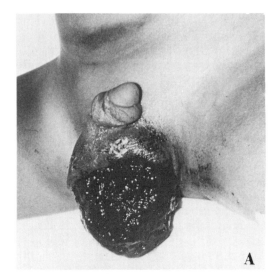

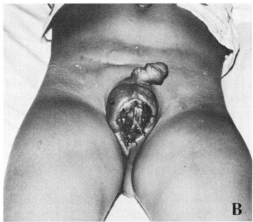

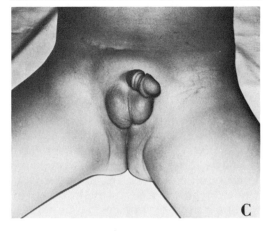

Figure 3-10. A, Scrotal hematoma with scrotal skin slough and subcutaneous hematoma of perineum and thighs in a four year old with severe Factor VIII deficiency. B, Healing of skin slough and C, eventual complete recovery without testicular involvement.

growth and weight problems, acne, and all other problems common to adolescents. The emotional trauma and strain of normal adolescence may be greatly complicated by the presence of hemophilia or any other chronic, disabling problem. Thus, adolescent hemophiliacs need consistent guidance and counseling as well as medical care directed not only toward bleeding problems but toward general growth problems common to this age.

Because these adolescent patients are usually physically active, hemarthroses and soft tissue hemorrhages continue to be annoying and painful problems. Inadequate care of recurrent hemarthroses during this age period may result in the initiation of permanent, progressive, degenerative arthropathy.

Hemarthroses of knees, ankles, or elbows should be treated by concentrate administration, joint aspiration, rest, and brief immobilization. When synovitis is extensive, as manifested by synovial thickening, increased surface temperature, and considerable effusion, anti-inflammatory medications may be helpful. Use of these drugs is described later in this chapter. Additional information about the management of specific joint complaints is found in Chapter 6.

Soft tissue hemorrhages in the adolescent often occur in the deep muscular tissue and below fascial planes (Fig. 3-11). Although these hemorrhages are usually not life threatening, they should be vigorously treated because of the severe

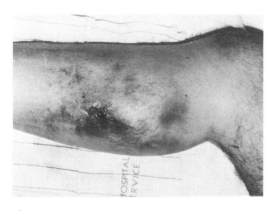

Figure 3-11. Hematoma of the calf with skin necrosis.

pain, the possible peripheral neuropathy, and the subsequent muscle fibrosis. Ultrasound may hasten the resolution of such hemorrhages.

Retroperitoneal or *iliopsoas* hemorrhage deserves special comment because of the frequency with which it occurs and the management problems it presents. The hemorrhage may mimic acute appendicitis or other acute surgical abdominal conditions but nausea and vomiting are not as severe or persistent. Diagnostic features may include: (1) pain in the groin, in the right or left lower quadrant, or radiating into the scrotal area; (2) swelling may be palpable; (3) rebound tenderness; or (4) decreased peristalsis. The leg on the affected side is held in hip flexion. Attempted hip extension is painful, however, rotation is essentially pain free. Paresthesia or hyperesthesia may be present in the cutaneous areas served by the genitofemoral nerve, the lateral femoral cutaneous nerve, and/or the sensory branches of the femoral nerve itself. Paresis of the quadriceps femoris muscle group may be present.

When the symptoms are mild in degree, daily concentrate administration is provided. Bedrest for a two to three day period is indicated with ambulation progressing slowly from crutch usage to full weight bearing. Strenuous physical activity is discouraged for two to three months. Management of severe iliopsoas hemorrhage includes bedrest in the position of comfort, adequate analgesics, and infusion of plasma products to achieve 50 percent levels for several days or weeks. Dosages may be reduced to attain levels of 20 to 30 percent when exercise and gradual ambulation are instituted. Further details are found in Chapter 6.

MANAGEMENT OF THE ADULT HEMOPHILIAC

General Health Care

Medical management of the adult hemophiliac must stress maintenance of good general health, early detection of medical problems not related to hemophilia, and appropriate treatment for hemophilia and its related problems. As hematologic management of the disease improves, the life span of the adult with hemophilia can more closely approach that of the normal male. However, the older hemophiliacs will face the same risks as the normal population of suffering degenerative cardiovascular problems, carcinoma, and other diseases of the aging. A complete medical examination including tests of liver and renal function and appropriate radiographs of the chest and major joints are performed annually. The importance of weight control is emphasized by the physician to the patient. Both the patient and the physician should constantly remember that the hemophiliac is not immune to other diseases; management of bleeding problems does not obviate the need for comprehensive medical care. An ongoing, close relationship with one physician is emphasized.

Management of Specific Problems

Chronic, severe, *degenerative arthritis* is the most frequent problem confronting the physician who manages the care of adult hemophiliacs. Seventy-five percent of hemophilic adults have one or more affected joints. The synovial and joint changes initiated by recurrent hemarthroses produce the disabling arthropathy characterized by morning stiffness and positional gelling, variable joint pain, limitation of joint motion, muscle atrophy, and finally fibrous ankylosis.

Anti-inflammatory drugs may be employed but are of limited usefulness. These include indomethacin, 25 mg three times daily, or prednisone for short, 10 day courses. The latter is more useful when synovitis is prominent. Oral analgesics such as acetaminophen or propoxyphene, alone or in combination, may reduce the discomfort to a tolerable level. Exercise and assistive orthopedic devices may further decrease some complaints.

The hemophilic adult patient may be helped to endure his more or less chronic joint discomfort by emotional support from the physician and the therapist and the understanding that toleration of some pain and discomfort is preferable to increased analgesic medication.

Hepatitis or posthepatic cirrhosis are caused by the serum hepatitis virus (SH or MS2 or hepatitis B virus) transmitted through pooled plasma products prepared from large numbers of donors. Approximately 1.3 cases of clinical hepatitis per 100 patients are found each year at Orthopaedic Hospital. The incidence of hepatitis can be reduced by using low-risk, single donor cryoprecipitate or fresh frozen plasma for patients who receive treatment infrequently.

Following an incubation period of 15 days to 6 months, the usually benign course which may be anicteric proceeds to apparent clinical recovery. Chronic hepatitis with hepatic failure and cirrhosis is rare. The prognosis for recovery is excellent with conservative management. If bleeding problems occur during the course of hepatitis, the usual treatment is given.

Following an occurrence of hepatitis, the patient is instructed to avoid contact with known hepatotoxic drugs and chemicals including dry cleaning chemicals and excessive alcohol intake. Liver function is periodically rechecked following hepatitis on a six month or yearly basis, assuming the patient is asymptomatic. Radiographic studies of the esophagus or endoscopic studies of the esophagus or stomach may be indicated when symptoms and signs of bleeding from the upper intestinal tract occur.

Gastrointestinal tract complaints may be acute or chronic and may or may not be hemorrhagic in nature. In general, bleeding from the gastrointestinal tract is not assumed only on the basis of hemophilia. Other sources of pathology such as ulcer, colitis, carcinoma, and polyps are investigated and treated appropriately. Gastrointestinal hemorrhage demands vigorous treatment with blood replacement, plasma concentrate administered every 8 to 12 hours to attain a 50 percent level, and diagnostic tests to determine the source of the bleeding. Diagnostic tests may include both radiographic and endoscopic examination of the gastrointestinal tract. Gastrointestinal hemorrhage may produce massive, sudden blood loss with resulting hypovolemic shock. Patients are hospitalized for careful observation until the bleeding is controlled and its source determined.

A *peptic ulcer* may be manifested by hematemesis or melena. Radiologic studies are performed when the hemorrhage is controlled. Conservative treatment of peptic ulcer consisting of a bland or soft diet, and antispasmodic and antacid medication may be effective in promoting ulcer healing with cessation of hemorrhage. If these measures prove ineffective and the hemorrhaging continues, surgery may be required as it is for the nonhemophilic patient for control of ulcer bleeding. When a hemophilic patient enters the hospital with sudden and profuse gastrointestinal bleeding, a general surgeon is included promptly in the treatment team so that care may be shared by the internist and the surgeon as the patient's course indicates.

The signs and symptoms of acute appendicitis may be mimicked by right-sided retroperitoneal or iliopsoas hemorrhage. Occasionally, immediate diagnosis is not possible and the patient is managed conservatively with intravenous fluids, intravenous antibiotics, and appropriate factor replacement to a surgical level in case a laparotomy is necessary. The patient should be given nothing by mouth during this observation period. Frequent monitoring should include white blood counts with differential, urinalyses, and radiographs of the abdomen and chest to establish a more precise diagnosis. Usually an increase in white blood count combined with a "left shift" is more pronounced with acute appendicitis than with retroperitoneal bleeding. Intraperitoneal bleeding, particularly into the mesentery, may produce a picture almost identical with acute appendicitis; laparotomy is necessary on rare occasions to determine which condition is present. During the period of observation, the patient should

receive maximum treatment for possible appendicitis with impending perforation as well as for a major bleeding episode.

Gastroenteritis with severe vomiting and diarrhea may provoke gastrointestinal bleeding. Other gastrointestinal tract hemorrhages may include: (1) intramural hemorrhage, particularly of the duodenum, secondary to abdominal trauma; (2) mesenteric hematoma; (3) bleeding from polyps in the colon; and (4) bleeding from hemorrhoids or anal or rectal fissures.

A 15½ year old with severe classic hemophilia had a three day history of increasingly severe diarrhea, vomiting, intermittent burning, and abdominal pain. On admission to the hospital he demonstrated periumbilical tenderness without evidence of an intra-abdominal mass or organomegaly. Abnormal findings in the terminal ilium and cecum were described following upper gastrointestinal radiography with and without the introduction of barium. The radiographic findings were consistent with either terminal ileitis or an extrinsic pressure defect. The patient was treated conservatively with intravenous fluids, antispasmodic medication, and Factor VIII concentrate. He gradually improved, was instructed to follow a bland diet at home, and was to return for further investigation if the symptoms recurred. No recurrence was noted.

"Essential" hypertension has an apparent increased incidence among adult hemophiliacs. Medical control is aggressive. Other causes of hypertension are considered and investigated.

Endocrine diseases are explored carefully and managed as in nonhemophilic patients. When possible, *diabetes mellitus* is controlled by dietary measures. When control is not effected by this measure, insulin may be administered in the usual dosage and manner. Insulin administration does not cause significant hematoma formation, hence, prior infusion of plasma products is not indicated.

Thyroid disorders, i.e., goiter, hyperthyroidism or hypothyroidism, are treated in the nonhemophilic manner. Possibly, a marked hyperthyroid state, with increased metabolism, may alter the biokinetics of Factor VIII or IX.

Renal problems may arise as separate entities or may result from repeated episodes of hematuria with secondary obstructive uropathy.

At age 42, a patient with known severe classic hemophilia was discovered to have hypertension. His history throughout childhood and youth was one of multiple episodes of joint hemorrhage, soft tissue hemorrhage, and frequent bouts of hematuria. Because of his severe arthritic problems, over the years he had taken a number of medications including both phenylbutazone and indomethacin. Following the discovery of hypertension, he was found to have impaired kidney function with markedly decreased creatinine clearance, elevated blood urea nitrogen, and elevated serum creatinine. Infusion renograms as well as radioisotope renal scan studies revealed decreased renal function bilaterally with a large defect in the right lower pole of the right kidney. His hypertension is moderately well controlled by medication; his creatinine clearance and blood urea nitrogen values fluctuate from time to time but have not approached normal. Currently, he is unable to work because of fatigue, headache, and visual problems which appear to have no organic basis. His provisional diagnosis of the renal problem is chronic pyelonephritis with compromised kidney function and severe hemophilia A.

Occasional renal calculi are recognized and treated aggressively because they may precipitate repeated bouts of kidney bleeding. Experience with prostatectomy is quite limited but as the patient group grows older, benign prostatic hypertrophy, or prostatic carcinoma will certainly show an increased incidence because of increasing age.

ROUTINE SURGICAL MANAGEMENT

Preoperative Evaluation

A complete hematologic diagnosis, including tests for inhibitors to Factor VIII or IX, is mandatory before surgery is contemplated. The availability of experienced and competent hematologic supervision is essential for successful surgery; *surgery should not be undertaken on hemophiliacs except in extreme life-threatening circumstances unless such consultation is immediately available.* When facilities are not adequate, it is wiser to transport the hemophilic patient to a center with an experienced hematologist and appropriate laboratory facilities rather than delay or procrastinate when surgery seems probable or even possible. Before surgery is undertaken, the estimated amounts of blood products (cryoprecipitate, whole blood, plasma concentrates) should be stockpiled so that adequate supplies are available for the surgical and convalescent periods.

A complete medical preoperative evaluation includes a physical examination, an electrocardiograph, a chest X-ray, and biochemical tests of liver and renal function.

General Guidelines
for Surgical/Hematologic Management

Prophylactic or elective surgery should *not* be undertaken in Factor IX patients until the thromboembolic problems associated with Factor IX concentrate can be prevented. The patient's Factor VIII or IX level is raised to 100 percent levels immediately prior to surgery and is maintained at minimal daily levels of 30 percent during the healing period, which varies with the type of surgery. Administration of concentrate or plasma products is continued for a minimum of 10 to 14 days. Following orthopedic surgery, replacement therapy is administered during the convalescent period when mobilization and exercise are initiated. If extensive whole blood replacement is necessary during or after a major surgical procedure, additional concentrate or cryoprecipitate is required as part of the blood replacement. Fever, infection, or other elevated metabolic demands upon the body increase the consumption of Factor VIII or IX in the postoperative period. When fever, infection, or rapid bleeding cause increased consumption and turnover of these plasma factors, doses of plasma concentrates are increased not only in total amount, but also in frequency of administration. Thus, it may be necessary to administer AHF concentrate on an every 6 hour or every 8 hour basis instead of every 12 hours because of the shortened half-life.

General Postconvalescent Care

During the convalescent period, the patient ambulates as soon as possible depending upon the nature of the surgery; the usual precautions are taken to avoid thromboembolic phenomena. Mobilization of nonaffected extremities is important when multiple arthritic manifestations are present. Prophylactic antibiotics are not indicated unless the possibility of a wound hematoma or other deep hematoma exists. Care is taken to assure that the patient receives adequate analgesic medication during the postoperative period keeping in mind his prior exposure to analgesics.

4

NURSING CARE

Enid F. Eckert

OUTPATIENT MANAGEMENT

General Information

Outpatient management is the preferred approach to the treatment of routine non-life threatening hemorrhages; this approach is safe, costs less than hospitalization, and is less disruptive to the daily life of the patient. The patients will seek treatment more readily when they know they will be treated *effectively* and efficiently with minimal delay and without hospitalization.

Following diagnosis of the type and severity of hemophilia, the hematologist calculates dosages of plasma products for each patient for minor and major bleeding episodes based upon his body weight. (Complete information is contained in Chapter 2 about the diagnosis and the types of hemophilia as well as the plasma products used in treatment.) A record is maintained in the treatment area, separate from the patient's outpatient chart, which indicates the dosage information as well as the patient's name, type and severity of hemophilia, blood type, birthdate, and hospital identification number. Treatment information documented on this record includes: date, site, and duration of bleeding episodes; type and amounts of plasma products administered; other treatment such as prescribed medication, joint aspiration, and so forth. (Figs. 4-1 and 4-2).

A hemophilic patient seeking treatment for hemorrhages or other complaints comes without prior appointment to the outpatient treatment room. The registered nurse in charge of the treatment room evaluates the complaint and gives treatment if the problem is a routine one. She refers emergency or extraordinary hemorrhagic or medical problems to a Hemophilia Center physician for management. Additionally, there is a specific daily time when patients can be examined by a Center physician for unresolved hemorrhages or ailments such as colds or influenza.

The treatment room nurse is skilled in venipuncture and is trained in evaluating bleeding problems as well as general health assessment. Pediatric or family nurse practitioner training would be extremely valuable for a nurse to function in this capacity.

The physician in charge must assume responsibility for carefully instructing the nurse about hemophilia and its management. It is the responsibility of the nurse, who has the most frequent contact with the patients, to listen carefully to their description of problems, symptoms, and anxieties. She should thoroughly explain all procedures and relay pertinent information to other appropriate staff members. Patients question freely their treatment and their condition and are given reasonable explanations.

Patient Education

Because we believe that all patients should know a great deal about their disease, all staff members participate in patient/parent education. Teaching occurs in the treatment room, in the outpatient clinics, in the physical therapy de-

NAME		OPD #	812 - RRNT-36749 B

PHYSICIAN'S ORDERS		PRESCRIPTIONS
DATE		DATE	

Figure 4-1. Outpatient Treatment Record.

partment, and literally wherever patients are seen or treated. All aspects of hemophilia and its impact on life are openly discussed including manifestations of the disease, indications for treatment, general health care, physical and recreational activities, the importance of routine ongoing preventive medical, orthopedic and dental care, family and genetic counseling, and vocational or educational guidance. Parental counseling stressing emphasis on normal childhood development is paramount. Family counseling and educational guidance information can be found in Chapters 11 and 12. Presurgical counseling is especially important so that the patient fully understands the procedure to be performed, the results to be expected, the inhospital course of management, and the specifics of convalescence.

Practical guidance aids parents in the physical protection of their young child. Examples include: padding the *inside* of pants and shirts to protect knees and elbows, moving furniture with sharp corners from the center of the room, avoiding toys with sharp or broken edges, placing protective cushioning on the corners of kitchen counter tops. A soft play sur-

NAME	# OF BOTTLES DISPENSED		OPD #	
				812 - RRNT-36749A

AREA OF BLEEDING	DATE		DATE		DATE		DATE		DATE		DATE		DATE		DATE		DATE		DATE	
	R	L	R	L	R	L	R	L	R	L	R	L	R	L	R	L	R	L	R	L
ELBOW																				
KNEE																				
SHOULDER																				
HIP																				
WRIST																				
ANKLE																				
HAND																				
FOOT																				
RETROPERITONEAL																				
BEHIND KNEE																				
FOREARM																				
CALF																				
OTHER AREAS (SPECIFY)																				
HEAD																				
NECK																				
THROAT																				
NOSE																				
MOUTH																				
FACE																				
INTESTINAL																				
URINARY																				
OTHER (SPECIFY)																				
HOW LONG HAVE YOU BEEN BLEEDING?																				
NAME OF CONCENTRATE USED																				
# OF BOTTLES USED																				
LOT #																				
# OF UNITS PER BOTTLE																				
MEDICATIONS PROBLEMS OR COMMENTS IF ANY-																				
SIGNATURE																				

OPD NO._____B/D

NAME.

HEMO TYPE_____LEVEL_____BLOOD TYPE_____

Figure 4-2. Plasma Products Administration Record.

face such as a lawn is preferable to a concrete yard. Floors should be carpeted for the same reason. Tricycles should be selected which have a low center of gravity and a wide axle between the rear wheels. Protective devices, such as helmets, are *discouraged* since these tend to differentiate the child from his peers. He should be allowed to play with normal children his own age. He should be subjected to the same rules, responsibilities, and discipline as other children. Emphasis is placed upon raising the hemophilic child as normally as possible.

Physical Facilities

The treatment room, located in the outpatient clinic building, is open five days per week; care is provided in the hospital emergency room at other times. The physical set-up of the treatment room includes space for examination table, comfortable chairs with footrests, a sink, and working space for the nurse. Equipment kept in an adjacent medicine room includes a variety of intravenous tubing and solutions, syringes, dressings and dressing trays, aspiration equipment, skin preparation materials, resuscitation equipment, antiseptics, culture and specimen tubes. A medicine drawer contains analgesics, antihistamines, and the usual emergency medications. Slings, prefabricated splints, crutches, and plaster are also kept in the area. The refrigerator and freezer for all plasma product storage is in this room. All plasma concentrates are refrigerated for storage; fresh-frozen plasma and cryoprecipitate are kept in a freezer at a temperature of −30°C. The weekly medical, pediatric, and orthopedic clinics are held in examination rooms adjacent to the treatment room and the coagulation laboratory.

Intravenous Administration Techniques

Because these patients are potential life-long consumers of intravenous plasma products, great care must be taken to preserve their veins. Developing rapport with and the confidence of infants and toddlers is vital since these children will be subjected to innumerable infusions. The parent is present at the time of treatment and physically cuddles the child during the infusion. Using the parent

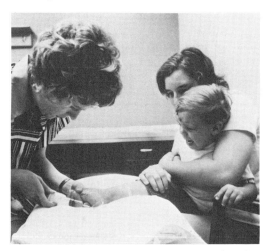

Figure 4-3. The child is held closely by mother during an infusion.

rather than a restraining board reduces the emotional anxiety of both the child and his parent at this potentially stressful time (Fig. 4-3). In this manner, children adapt quickly and without fear to the treatment procedure. Under no circumstances should the threat of infusion be used as a form of punishment; the occasional parent who tells his child to "behave or you will get a shot" should be re-educated promptly. As soon as the child develops some understanding, the treatment is explained simply to him as "the shot to make the hurt go away." (A detailed explanation of intravenous techniques appears as Appendix 1.)

General Guideline for Managing Bleeding Episodes

The earlier an episode is treated, the less pain and bleeding is likely to occur; hopefully, permanent crippling will also decrease. The more knowledgeable the patient and his family are about the disease, the greater are the chances that early treatment will be obtained. Patients can detect bleeding in joint and soft tissue areas before signs are apparent to an examiner. A relatively small dosage of concentrate at the first indication of bleeding will usually stop the hemorrhage quickly; then the patient can resume normal activities. If treatment is delayed, problems are compounded: larger amounts of concentrate are necessary, immobilization of the limb or entire body may be indicated, and absence from school or work will be increased. During treatment for a bleeding episode, the patient is given instruction about resting or immobilizing the bleeding area as well as comfortable positioning; about the use of crutches or splints and the resumption of normal activities; and about the need for additional dosages of concentrate as well as appointments to medical or orthopedic clinics.

Bleeding episodes are classified as minor or major. *Minor bleeding episodes* include those into the following areas as long as early treatment is instituted: (1) knee, ankle, shoulder, elbow, and wrist hemarthroses; (2) superficial soft tissue bleeding of the limbs; (3) nose, lip, tongue, or gum bleeding. Ordinarily, physician consultation is unnecessary; sufficient concentrate or cryoprecipitate is given to elevate the patient's factor level to 30 to 50 percent. Any large strawberry-like clots are removed from the mouth following the infusion.

For joint and soft tissue bleeding, the dosage is repeated in 24 hours if the hemorrhage does not resolve, i.e., continued acute pain, consistent swelling, and so forth. For nose, lip, gum, and tongue bleeding, a repeat infusion is given in 24 hours even though further bleeding is not evident. The patient's diet is restricted to soft, cool foods for at least three days following mouth bleeding. Use of straws is prohibited during this period to avoid dislodging the formed clot. Antifibrinolytic drugs such as epsilon-amino-caproic acid may be prescribed by the physician if bleeding is persistent. Slight oozing may occur when deciduous teeth are shed. Generally, pressure applied to the gum for a short time will stop the bleeding; concentrate is not needed unless the oozing is persistent.

Major bleeding episodes include potentially life-threatening hemorrhages as well as those into other vital areas: (1) head, neck, throat, kidney, intestinal, retroperitoneal, iliopsoas, hip joint, and abdominal area bleeding; (2) deep muscle bleeding especially into calf, hamstring, or forearm sites; (3) hemarthrosis which is unresolved or in which treatment was delayed. Concentrate or cryoprecipitate is infused to attain 50 percent factor levels. Dosages are repeated every 12 to 24 hours depending upon the location and the severity of the problem. Physician examination is essential.

Detailed management of intracranial, oropharyngeal, gastrointestinal, retroperitoneal, and iliopsoas hemorrhages is found in Chapter 3. However, certain comments will aid in the practical examination and management of specific problems.

HEAD TRAUMA. Infusion of plasma products is essential with any history of trauma to the head even though bleeding symptoms may be absent. When neurologic signs are absent, the patient may return home following concentrate or cryoprecipitate administration and physician examination. However, family members are thoroughly instructed to observe the patient for adverse symptoms such as headache, dizziness, dilated or unequal pupils, drowsiness, nausea, vomiting, or confusion. Detection of any of these symptoms necessitates an immediate return to the hospital.

THROAT HEMORRHAGE. Often, throat bleeding results from tonsillar infection although small children may injure the throat by poking hard or pointed objects into the posterior oral cavity. With neck hemorrhages, anterior or lateral swelling may be apparent with or without difficulty in swallowing or breathing. When bleeding is not severe, the patient returns home following physician examination and the initial concentrate administration. Family members are instructed to observe for symptoms of respiratory distress. If throat bleeding is mistaken for mumps, the consequences may be disastrous.

KIDNEY BLEEDING. Blood in the urine may appear pink, dark red, or brownish; clots may be present. Concentrate or cryoprecipitate is administered. Fluid intake of 150 to 200 ml per hour and bedrest are advised until the urine is straw colored. Frequently, recurring or slowly resolving hematuria necessitates close follow-up by the physician as further diagnostic tests may be indicated. Antifibrinolytic drugs such as epsilon-amino-caproic acid are contraindicated.

ABDOMINAL WALL HEMORRHAGES. Daily concentrate or cryoprecipitate is administered until the hemorrhage resolves. Rib fracture or splenic rupture should be ruled out. Hospitalization will be necessary if bleeding is severe. By falling against the handlebars of tricycles, toddlers may sustain abdominal or chest wall hemorrhages.

DEEP MUSCLE BLEEDING. Hemorrhage into muscular areas, particularly flexor locations, can be quite extensive and dissect through tissue planes. Aspiration is impossible because the hemorrhage is not confined to an isolated area; concentrate is infused daily for several consecutive days. Early detection of peripheral nerve involvement is important to prevent long-term or permanent injury. Details of splinting and other follow-up care of certain muscle hemorrhages are covered in Chapter 6.

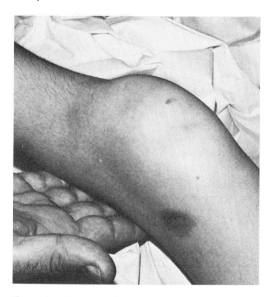

Figure 4-4. Extensive hemarthrosis of the knee.

Extensive Hemarthroses. Aspiration may be employed by the resident, house staff, or Center physician when a patient's knee, elbow, or ankle is marked by swelling or exquisite pain (Fig. 4-4). Short-term effects of arthrocentesis are a more rapid return to normal function and relief of pain; long-term effects may be a reduction of the cartilaginous destruction attributed to the presence of the bloody effusion. Plasma factor levels are elevated to 50 percent at the time of the arthrocentesis and to 20 percent on the fourth or fifth postaspiration day. The skin over the joint to be aspirated is prepared in a routine preoperative manner; a local anesthetic is injected at the site of needle insertion into the joint. The aspiration needle is 15 or 18 gauge. Since immediate pain relief usually follows arthrocentesis, routine use of narcotics for control of pain is unnecessary.

Elastic bandages are applied at completion of the aspiration. The joint is immobilized for 24 hours as described in Chapter 6. When the knee or the ankle is aspirated, the patient uses crutches for at least 24 hours without bearing weight on the aspirated limb. The crutches are gradually discontinued as soon as weight bearing can occur without discomfort.

THE HOME TRANSFUSION PROGRAM

This program provides the most efficient method to immediately treat suspected bleeding episodes. The program began in 1968 with 12 participants and now has 150. Patients, parents, or other family members are taught to evaluate different types of bleeding episodes and to administer concentrate at home at the first sign of hemorrhage Concentrate is stored in the home refrigerator or transported in an iced cooler during vacations or traveling. This Center does not dispense cryoprecipitate for home use because of storage and transportation problems as well as the frequency of allergic reactions. Other centers in the United States and England have used cryoprecipitate on a self-infusion program.[1,2,3]

Patient Selection

Patient selection is based on the following criteria: ability and desire of the patient to participate, clearance by the Center physician, and frequency of bleeding episodes. Patients who seldom incur hemorrhages are poor candidates because they tend to forget the instructions and technical procedures during the intervals between hemorrhages. Also excluded are patients with medical complications such as presence of an inhibitor or severe allergic reactions to plasma products.

The child by the age of four to five years, generally has developed easily accessible veins, accepts venipuncture as a "matter of fact," and understands the reasons why treatment is necessary. At this age, parents are instructed in the procedure of preparing and administering concentrate to their child. When the child is nine or ten years old, he can often perform his own venipuncture successfully, but at this age he has difficulty with abstract aspects of the procedure. For this reason, further instruction is generally delayed until the child is approximately 12 to 13 years of age.

Patient Instruction

All instruction is conducted on an individual basis with the patient advancing at his own rate. The total instruction period varies from 5 to 20 hours. Teaching is divided into two parts: technical and theoretical.

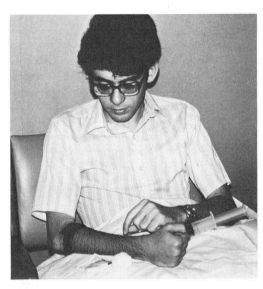

Figure 4-5. Self-administration of concentrate (syringe method).

TECHNICAL INSTRUCTION. The patient or parent is taught to prepare and administer the concentrates by both drip and syringe methods (Fig. 4-5). (The volume of some reconstituted concentrates is too great to administer by syringe method when several bottles are used at one time.) When all procedures are performed safely and independently by the patient under nurse supervision, written instructions are provided as sources of reference. (See Appendix 2, Home Transfusion Instructions.)

Patients and parents are advised of the potential hepatitis danger from handling these products. If the parent administering the concentrate accidentally stabs himself with a used needle, he is told to promote bleeding of the stab wound, and then to wash thoroughly with soap and water. Skin to mouth contact with spilled concentrate also poses a hepatitis source if the skin and the work area are not thoroughly cleansed after completion of the procedure.

THEORETICAL INSTRUCTION. All hemophilic patients should become knowledgeable about their disease. This knowledge is doubly important for those on the self-transfusion program. Patients learn to assess the severity of a bleeding episode and to differentiate symptoms which are potentially dangerous or crippling or require the attention of a physician (Fig. 4-6). Dosage information is provided for minor and major categories of bleeding episodes along with indications for repeating the concentrate dosage. When episodes do not respond following two administrations of concentrate, patients must return to the Center. Mild hemorrhages into hip, groin, retroperitoneal, calf, or forearm areas as well as kidney bleeding are supervised through daily telephone contact until the hemorrhage has resolved. Following any trauma to the head or hemorrhage into the neck, patients must return to the Center.

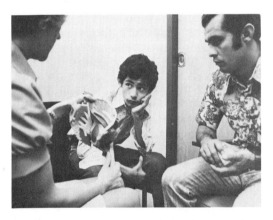

Figure 4-6. Visual aids are used to explain to patient and father the location of internal hemorrhages.

Materials and Equipment

Following satisfactory completion of the instruction sessions, the dispensed supplies include concentrate, intravenous tubing, syringes, needles, tourniquet, and alcohol sponges. Individualized dosage instruction sheets are provided (Appendix 2) as well as a supply of bleeding episode record forms which are identical to those maintained in the out-patient department. (See Fig. 4-2.) Patients are guided in appropriate storage of the concentrate and other supplies as well as disposal of used equipment and empty bottles.

Routine Follow-Up

Each participant in the home transfusion program records every administration of concentrate on the proper form and furnishes this record to the Center nurse when additional concentrate or supplies are required. Failure to provide these administration records results in the discontinuation from the home program. The nurse reviews these records and helps the patient with problems or questions which may arise.

Recurrent bleeding problems into a specific joint are referred to the orthopedic clinic. Body weights are obtained every six months to determine that the recommended concentrate dosages are sufficient; this factor is especially important for growing children. Obesity should be avoided since excess weight will compound joint problems. Every home transfusion participant has annual physical and orthopedic examinations as well as range of motion testing and radiographic evaluation. Standard form letters are given to those patients who are travelling away from the Center to explain the supplies of concentrate and the administration equipment which the patient carries.

Patients are removed from the self-transfusion program whenever medical problems develop, such as an inhibitor or allergic responses to concentrate. Evidence of drug abuse or addiction, and failure to comply with instructions are also grounds for removal from the home program.

Advantages of the home program include: (1) prompt treatment of bleeding; (2) reduced pain; (3) rapid resolution of hemorrhage and return to normal activities; (4) decreased transportation costs to and from the hospital; (5) minimal time lost from school or work. For example, one family in a one year period traveled 10,000 miles between hospital and home prior to participating in a home transfusion program.

In another case, one child averaged nine visits per month to the hospital before beginning home transfusions. Delays of several hours occurred between the onset of bleeding and treatment and the patient suffered greatly from pain. His return to normal daily activities was often delayed two to three days and he was absent from school 50 percent of the time. Since participating in the home transfusion program he has been absent an average of only three days of school per month.

INPATIENT MANAGEMENT

Patients are hospitalized for severe hemorrhages which cannot be managed safely out of the hospital, for emergency or elective surgery, for intensive physical therapy programs, and for *any* medical problem ordinarily requiring hospitalization. Direct nursing care of the hospitalized patient is given by the nursing staff of the hospital unit with the Center nurse providing necessary coordination. The unit staff is informed about hemophilia in general, and about a specific patient including his anxieties, expectations, and idiosyncracies as well as his immediate medical or physical problems and helpful nursing measures. In-service education includes instruction about correct preparation and administration of concentrates and cryoprecipitates when nurses are unfamiliar with these medications.

Unit nursing personnel are reminded to give special consideration to the hemophilic patient regarding his use of pain medication. Because he may need to use pain medication frequently as an outpatient he often requires more narcotics than the average patient when he is hospitalized with severe pain. Nurses tend to become concerned about patients with chronic complaints of pain and fear that the patient is becoming addicted to narcotics. The nurse should discuss these concerns with the patient's physician, not with the patient. The physician's recommendations should be followed. Medication can be safely administered by the intramuscular route when the patient is being transfused with concentrate on a daily basis; however, subcutaneous injections are preferable whenever possible.

Patients on the home transfusion program are allowed to start their own infusions during hospitalizations. They are usually successful with the first venipuncture, while nurses and physicians may attempt venipuncture several times before success is achieved.

Planning for hospital discharge assures a smooth transition from hospital to home. The following questions are considered: Is equipment such as a hospital bed, a walker, or a commode needed in the home? Can the patient transfer from bed to chair or chair to car? Can the patient drive? Can he manage self-infusion? If he is not on the home transfusion program, how will he transport himself to the hospital if he needs concentrate or other follow-up care? When can he return to work or school? A visit to the patient's home prior to discharge will allow an evaluation of the situation. A second visit may be necessary following discharge if problems become apparent.

COMMUNITY RESOURCES

The most frequently contacted community institutions are the schools attended by our patients. The Center staff makes telephone or personal contact when a child enters a new school and as needed during the school year. School personnel may express anxiety about hemophilic students attending regular school. This attitude is usually due to lack of knowledge about the disease and limited exposure to such students. They are assured that the hemophilic child will not bleed severely from small cuts since these are managed ordinarily as are the cuts of nonhemophilic children. They are educated about the disease and its treatment and advised about the occasional physical limitations imposed upon a child during a bleeding episode. Periodic need for crutches or other assistive devices is explained as are the reasons for sporadic absences.

The school nurse receives specific information about the management of certain problems such as nosebleeds and about the problems that demand parental notification. Particular emphasis is placed on the potentially life-threatening aspect of any head injury and the importance of promptly alerting the parent so the child can be transported to the Center for examination and treatment. Coordination between the child's physical education teacher and Center personnel, particularly the physical therapist, is important to establish appropriate physical activity levels. School personnel are encouraged to contact Center personnel whenever necessary.

SUMMARY

Outpatient management of routine nonlife-threatening hemorrhages can be provided effectively, efficiently, and economically. The nurse should have knowledge of location and function of muscles and location of nerves and blood vessels so that adequate assessment can be made of motor and sensory impairment when soft tissue hemorrhages are present. She should obtain a detailed history of each bleeding episode keeping in mind the possibility of fracture when trauma has occurred. The nurse should recognize other existing medical problems so that she can refer the patient to the physician.

Follow-up care is an essential element

of management of these patients and should include thorough patient/parent education. The home transfusion program provides additional benefits by reducing outpatient visits and long waiting periods between hemorrhage and treatment. Thus, the patient is allowed greater freedom to lead a more normal, fulfilling life.

REFERENCES

1. Rabiner, S. F., and Telfer, M. D.: Home transfusion for patients with hemophilia A. New Engl. J. Med. 283:1011, 1970.
2. Le Quesne, B., Maragaki, D., Britten, M., and Dormandy, K.: Home treatment for patients with hemophilia. Lancet 2:507, 1974.
3. Van Eys, J., Agle, D., Hilgartner, M., and Lazerson, J.: Home Therapy for Hemophilia. New York, National Hemophilia Foundation, 1974.

5

RADIOLOGIC EVALUATION

R. R. Schreiber

Bleeding into various areas of the body results in changes visible on roentgenograms in many instances. Ordinary roentgen techniques are usually sufficient for radiologic evaluation of the affected areas. The term "hemophilic arthropathy" is used to refer to the changes which develop in joints after repeated episodes of intra-articular bleeding in hemophiliacs.

There is no difference in the changes seen radiologically in hemophilia A and B. The extent of the arthropathy increases with the severity of the hemophilia.[1]

HEMORRHAGE IN NONMUSCULOSKELETAL AREAS

Bleeding into the kidneys may be shown by filling defects in the urinary drainage system at some point, obstruction to drainage, or total (temporary) shutdown of a kidney as judged on intravenous urography. Encroachment on the lumen of part of the gut can be shown by barium examination of the involved area. Extremely gentle or even no palpation should be used in the gastrointestinal examination on a hemophiliac with recent gastrointestinal bleeding for fear of dislodging a clot. Erect and recumbent positions with rotation of the patient usually suffice to show the anatomy. From a practical standpoint, precise localization of a leaking vessel in the intestinal tract is not usually necessary as the bleeding usually is controlled by nonsurgical management. Demonstration of an ulcer may be sought when symptoms and signs point to such a diagnosis.

MUSCULOSKELETAL HEMORRHAGE EVALUATION

Hemorrhage in soft tissues will result in swelling and obscuration of the usual soft tissue planes. Bulging of the psoas outline is frequently seen in retroperitoneal bleeding. The resulting fullness here may persist, even with clinical resolution, while in most other areas the fullness eventually disappears.

Bleeding into joints results in changes well depicted on routine roentgenograms, particularly in the areas most commonly affected: knees, ankles, elbows. The initial finding is joint capsule distention. In the knee, this is best shown by distention of the suprapatellar pouch. In the elbow, this is best shown by a positive fat pad sign in lateral view (appearance of and posterior displacement of the radiolucent stripe of the subsynovial fat in the posterior joint capsule at the olecranon fossa). In the ankle, capsular distention is shown by generalized fullness centered on the ankle joint. Enlargement of the medial hip joint space ("F-T" or femur-tear drop distance) is the most sensitive indicator of abnormality of the hip joint. The distention of any joint capsule may indicate either increased intra-articular fluid (blood, synovia, pus) or thickening of any part of or all of the capsule wall as from synovitis. If the blood is completely resorbed and synovitis does not ensue, the joint findings roentgenologically will return to normal.

In the knee, change in the joint space or cartilage space between bones is of use chiefly in the direction of decrease. Lack of resorption of blood will result in synovitis which can produce a series of changes in time. Narrowing of the joint space or joint cartilage indicates some destruction of the cartilage, the degree of narrowing reflecting the degree of destruction.

A typical sequence of events in an involved joint of a hemophiliac will be described, using the knee as an example: Bleeding into the joint will produce capsular distention. With repeated episodes of bleeding, sooner or later synovitis will be set up. Decreased activity results in some atrophy of muscle mass in the region of the knee. The capsular tissues and joint capsule are somewhat more prominent, probably not on the basis of hemosiderosis in the usual case. Hyperemia plus decreased use of the joint produce osteoporosis. With time, small erosions appear around the edges of the joint, off the articular surfaces, the cartilage space becomes narrow, and subchondral articular bone develops irregularities. With progression of the process, cyst-like lucencies develop in the subchrondral bone. These lucencies really are cysts and represent one of the most typical findings in the arthropathy of hemophilia. These cysts usually develop earlier and are more irregular and numerous in size and distribution than those seen in other arthritides, especially in children. The cysts which present immediately adjacent to the joint probably originate from the joint proper, while cysts at a distance from the joint probably represent bleeding within the bone. The bones forming the joint gradually become deformed, showing flattening or erosion. Considerable sclerosis usually develops in the subchrondral bone. Marginal osteophytes develop and are often numerous. With eventual inactivity of the process, the bone density in general may be normal with eburnation and sclerosis persisting in the subchondral bone. The picture roentgenographically then will be not unlike that resulting from other types of arthritis. In children, the hyperemia frequently results in coarsening of the trabecular pattern in and accelerated

maturation of the epiphyses adjacent to the joint. Either overgrowth or undergrowth may be the result ultimately.

Bony ankylosis is extremely rare in hemophiliacs, despite the extensively involved and deformed joint surfaces in advanced cases. Most of the few cases of bony ankylosis shown in hemophiliacs have been in knees, ankles, and subtalar joints.

Contrast arthrography is not used routinely in evaluating a hemophilic joint.

CLASSIFICATIONS. Several classifications have been developed for grading hemophilic arthropathy. These classifications have been proposed by Konig (1892),[2] Caffey and Schlessinger (1940),[3] DePalma and Cotler (1956),[4] Jordan (1958),[5] Novikova (1960),[6] Ahlberg (1965),[1] and Wood and associates (1969).[7] The purpose of a classification is to evaluate the progression of the process and therapy. The classification of DePalma and Cotler is a four grade clinical-and-roentgenographic one. The classification of Wood and associates is based on the roentgen findings. This classification assigns point values to various roentgen findings and is shown in Table 5-1.

Table 5-1. Classification of roentgen findings[7]

Feature	Degree	Score
Periarticular soft tissues	Thickening	1
Calcification		1
Joint space	Narrowed	1
	Widened (effusion)	1
	Synovial thickening	1
Epiphyses	Enlarged	1
Bone density	Mild porosis	1
	Severe porosis	2
	Harris' lines	1
Erosions	Few (1–4)	1
	Many (over 4)	2
Cysts	Few (1–4)	1
	Many (over 4)	2
Osteoarthritis	Mild	1
	Severe	2

Specific Joints

In his study of 157 patients with hemophilia A and B, Ahlberg[1] found hemophilic arthropathy as follows: 172 knees, 145 elbows, 96 ankles, 28 shoulders, 20 wrists, and 13 hips. This analysis gives a typical distribution of joint involvement in hemophilia. The lower extremities are involved somewhat more than the upper, as shown by these figures.

KNEE. The general roentgen findings in the knee have been given previously. Figure 5-1 illustrates these findings. Enlargement of the intercondylar fossa of the distal femur is sometimes seen in hemophilia (Fig. 5-2). On occasion the distal end of the patella shows a squared-off appearance as seen in the lateral view. This finding may also be seen in

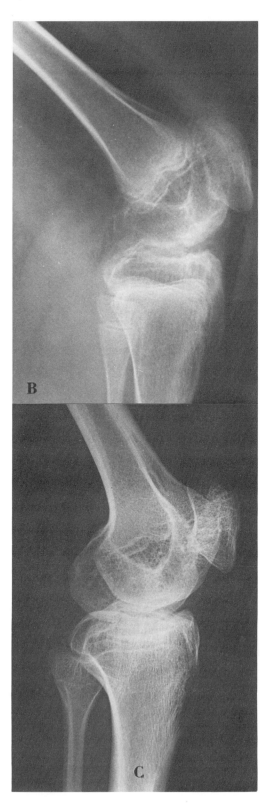

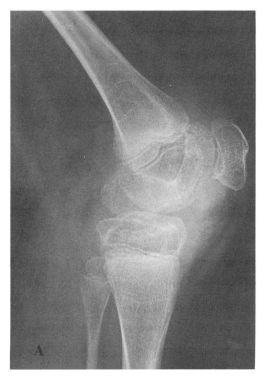

Figure 5-1. A, Ten-year-old male hemophiliac. The knee joint capsule is distended. Muscle masses are small, reflecting disuse. The joint spaces are a little narrow, particularly the patellofemoral where irregularities are developing in the subchondral cortices. There is generalized coarseness of trabecular pattern. B, The same patient at age 14. Subchondral articular cortices are more irregular. C, By age 20 the synovitis has become quiescent. Internal bony architecture shows good trabecular pattern and density. Subchondral articular cortices are more definite in outline and appear smoother.

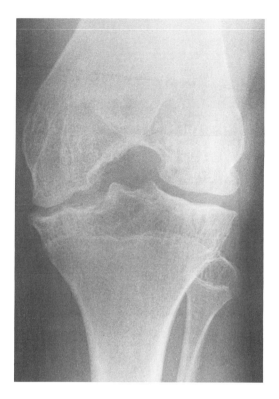

rheumatoid arthritis and rarely in normal patients. The patella may also show overgrowth (Fig. 5-3). The differential growth of the femoral condyles can result in genu varum or genu valgum.

Figure 5-2. Sixteen-year-old male with moderate hemophilic arthropathy. There are joint space narrowing medially, limited cyst formation, some marginal osteophytes, some enlargement of the intercondylar notch medially, and a persistently flexed attitude.

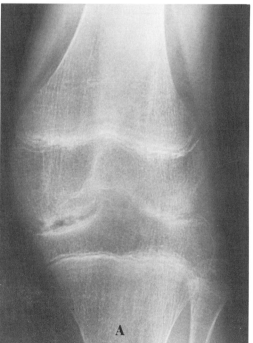

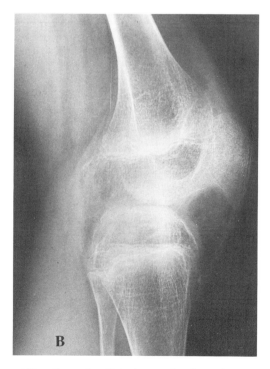

Figure 5-3. A, B, Twelve-year-old male with advanced hemophilic arthropathy. Note the paucity of muscle mass in the distal anterior thigh, the thin ligamentum patellae, the advanced narrowing of joint spaces with irregularity of subchondral cortices.

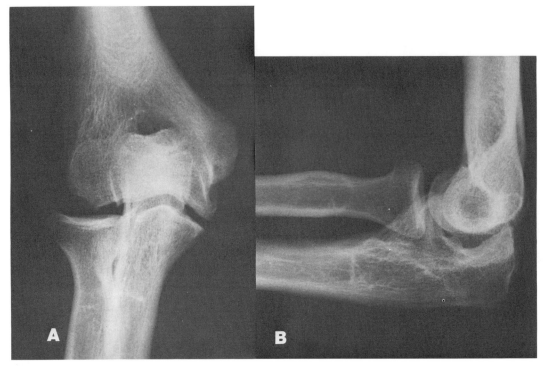

Figure 5-4. A, B, Thirty-seven-year-old male hemophiliac. The radial head is minimally broad, nowhere near as broad as some become. Erosions are present in the distal and lateral margins of the capitellum. Cysts are developing deep to the semilunar notch where there is some cortical erosion.

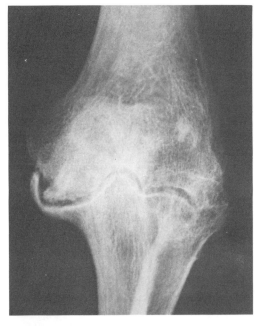

Figure 5-5. Forty-eight-year-old male with advanced hemophilic arthropathy of the radiohumeral and ulnohumeral joints. Joint spaces are narrow and the margins irregular to different degrees. The long standing erosion and reciprocal shaping of the ulna and the trochlea are noteworthy. Cysts are present.

ELBOW. The general findings in the elbow in hemophilic arthropathy have been described above. The subchondral cysts which are common in elbows involved with hemophilic arthropathy are much less common in other types of arthritis, especially in children. The semilunar notch often shows extensive erosion and broadening with severe involvement of this joint. The olecranon fossa may be enlarged. The head of the radius commonly shows overgrowth (Figs. 5-4 and 5-5).

ANKLE. The general findings described previously are applicable to the ankle. On occasion the top of the talus may show marked flattening. Collapse of the body of the talus has been described by Crock and Boni[8] and Ahlberg[1] (Figs. 5-6 and 5-7).

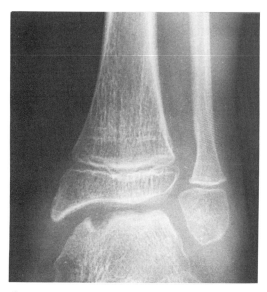

Figure 5-6. Six-year-old male with sizable erosions in the articular cortex of the talus and some narrowing of tibiotalar joint space as the early findings in his hemophilic arthropathy. Trabecular pattern is coarse.

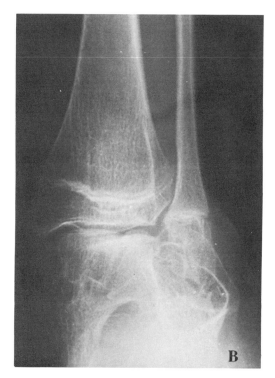

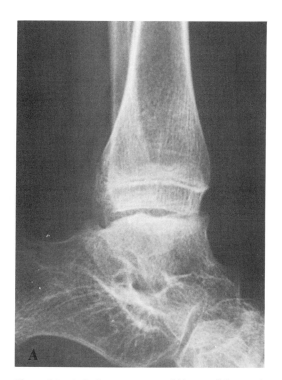

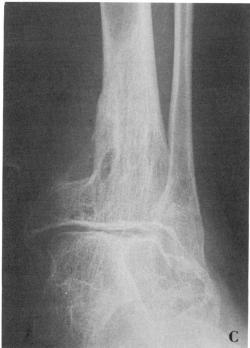

Figure 5-7. A, B, Fourteen-year-old hemophiliac with the top of the talus either eroded or collapsed to result in the altered contour shown in the lateral view. Joint space shows some narrowing. The contour of the subchondral cortex of the tibia is good. C, At age 18, the subchondral cortices are smoother, the joint space shows more uniform narrowing. A bizarre osteophyte is present on the tip of the medial malleolus. At least one cyst is present deep to the tibial joint cortex. The erosion centered in the distal medial tibial metaphyseal cortex probably represents the result of a pseudotumor which developed in a subperiosteal location.

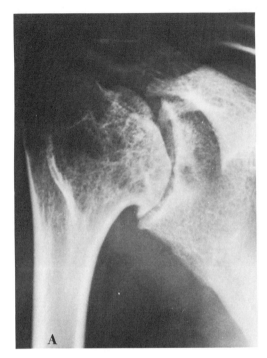
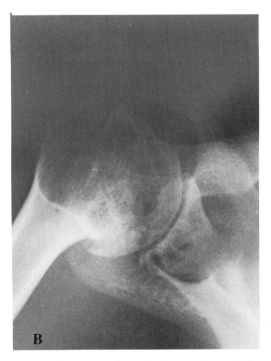

Figure 5-8. A, B, Anteroposterior and axillary views of the shoulder showing moderately advanced hemophilic arthropathy in a 26-year-old male.

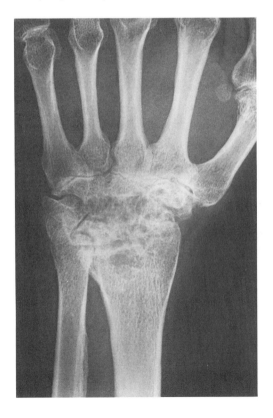

SHOULDER. The roentgen findings in the shoulder are as described previously for the general situation. Narrowing of the joint space, erosion, cysts, eburnation, and particularly osteophytes may be seen (Fig. 5-8).

HAND AND FOOT. The small joints of the hands and feet are infrequently involved (Fig. 5-9).

Figure 5-9. Advanced hemophilic arthropathy in the wrist of a 48-year-old male. Cysts are prominent. Arthropathy is also present in the fifth metacarpophalangeal joint, an uncommon location.

Hemophilic hip arthropathy can result in protrusio acetabuli.

Periosteal new bone formation secondary to subperiosteal bleeding is surprisingly uncommon in hemophilia. On occasion calcifications will develop following bleeding into soft tissues. On rare occasions a myositis ossificans-like picture may develop (Fig. 5-10). Subperiosteal new bone formation and callus are seen at fracture sites as in nonhemophiliacs. The healing process usually does not differ significantly from that in normals.

Pseudotumors

Pseudotumor is the name given to neoplasm-like changes seen in the bones of hemophiliacs. Pseudotumors are collections of blood which give the impression of being encapsulated and which clinically present as swellings and roentgenographically as neoplasm-like defects. The usual roentgen appearance is one of erosion as from pressure with fading away of the margins of the advancing area of lysis. The roentgen picture simulates that seen in aneurysmal bone cysts in nonhemophiliacs. In long bones, a typical picture would be an area of lysis centering in the cortex with expansion of periosteum and erosion of the underlying bone. Initially there is no reaction except lysis on the side of the bone. Eventually there is sclerosis along the margin of the lesion and the roentgen appearance becomes more benign. The subperiosteal new bone formed by stimulation and elevation of the periosteum will vary in amount with the speed of the process; there may be none if the process is rapid enough. In the hands and feet, the appearance is often that of expansion of an entire bone with fading away of margins. The sites most likely to be involved with a pseudotumor are the ilium, the femur and other long bones, hands and feet. The appearance in the hands and feet is suggestive of intraosseous origin. X-irradiation has been utilized in limited dosages in cases in which the process seemed life threatening, particularly in long bones (Fig. 5-11).

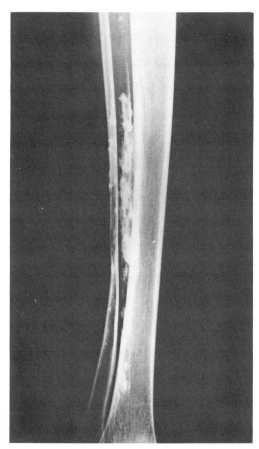

Figure 5-10. Calcifications in the soft tissues of the leg of a 10-year-old male with hemophilia. Soft tissue calcification and myositis ossificans are surprisingly rare following episodes of bleeding into soft tissues in hemophiliacs.

HIP. In the hip, the general changes described previously are applicable. In addition, a Legg-Perthes type of picture is seen on occasion prior to puberty. The flattening of the femoral capital epiphysis is likely not to be the typical anterolateral flattening seen in Legg-Perthes' disease.

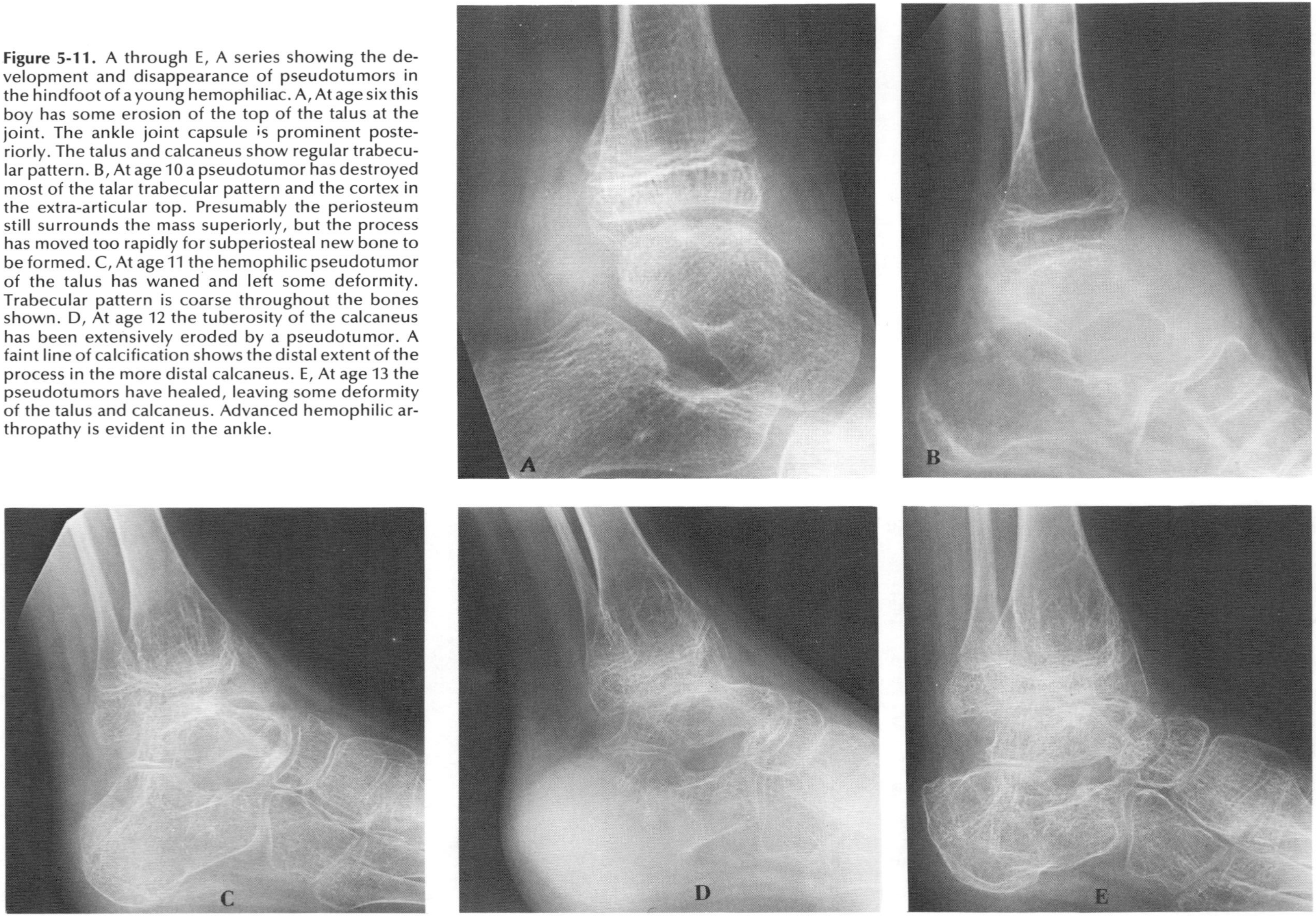

Figure 5-11. A through E, A series showing the development and disappearance of pseudotumors in the hindfoot of a young hemophiliac. A, At age six this boy has some erosion of the top of the talus at the joint. The ankle joint capsule is prominent posteriorly. The talus and calcaneus show regular trabecular pattern. B, At age 10 a pseudotumor has destroyed most of the talar trabecular pattern and the cortex in the extra-articular top. Presumably the periosteum still surrounds the mass superiorly, but the process has moved too rapidly for subperiosteal new bone to be formed. C, At age 11 the hemophilic pseudotumor of the talus has waned and left some deformity. Trabecular pattern is coarse throughout the bones shown. D, At age 12 the tuberosity of the calcaneus has been extensively eroded by a pseudotumor. A faint line of calcification shows the distal extent of the process in the more distal calcaneus. E, At age 13 the pseudotumors have healed, leaving some deformity of the talus and calcaneus. Advanced hemophilic arthropathy is evident in the ankle.

REFERENCES

1. Ahlberg, A.: Haemophilia in Sweden, VII. Incidence, treatment and prophylaxis of arthropathy and other musculoskeletal manifestations of haemophilia A and B. Acta Orthop. Scand. 77:5, 1965.
2. Konig, F.: Die Gelenkerkrankungen bei Blutern mit besonderer Berücksichtigung der Diagnose. Klin. Vorträge N.F. 36 (Chirurgie No. 11):233, 1892.
3. Caffey, J., and Schlessinger, E. R.: Certain effects of hemophilia on the growing skeleton. J. Pediatr. 16:549, 1940.
4. DePalma, A. F., and Cotler, J.: Hemophilic arthropathy. Clin. Orthopaed. 8:163, 1956.
5. Jordan, H. H.: *Hemophilic Arthropathies.* Charles C Thomas, Springfield, Ill., 1958.
6. Novikova, E. A.: Osteoarticular changes in hemophilia. Vestn. Rentgenol. Radiol. 2:13, 1960.
7. Wood, K., Omer, A., and Shaw, M. T.: Haemophilic arthropathy. Br. J. Radiol. 42:498, 1969.
8. Crock, H. V., and Boni, V.: The management of orthopaedic problems in haemophiliacs. A review of 21 cases. Br. J. Surg. 48:8, 1960.

6

COMMON MUSCULOSKELETAL PROBLEMS
AND THEIR MANAGEMENT

Donna C. Boone

BACKGROUND

The general philosophy of nonsurgical management of musculoskeletal problems was nurtured by Max Negri, M.D., who served for eight years as our senior orthopedic surgeon. The assistive devices described in this section were developed under his guidance and represented a dramatic departure from the traditional methods of bracing and relative immobilization utilized previously in the treatment of hemophilic arthropathy, as did his constant reiteration of the maxim of Hippocrates, "Exercise strengthens and inactivity wastes."

Four major aspects of this approach to treatment are: (1) the judicious treatment of each bleeding episode; (2) the initiation of exercise or other measures to normalize function and to decrease deformity; (3) the utilization of dynamic splints and other assistive devices for brief time intervals to support the limb or correct the deformity; and (4) a careful acute and a longitudinal evaluation of the musculoskeletal status of each patient.

GENERAL CONSIDERATION OF HEMOPHILIC ARTHROPATHY

Musculoskeletal residuals of hemorrhage, estimated to occur in 75 to 80 percent of the hemophilic population, present the most disabling consequences of these coagulation disorders. Hopefully, early diagnosis and treatment of each hemorrhage will reduce the crippling sequelae. Hemarthroses initiate charac-

teristically in childhood and tend to recur frequently and apparently spontaneously or unrelated to recognized trauma in those patients with severe disease. When patients with a mild or a moderate coagulation defect present with hemarthrosis, a history of injury can usually be obtained.

The hinged joints of the extremities are the most commonly affected while the hip and shoulder ball and socket joints are less frequently involved. However, some joints, even weight bearing ones, escape hemarthroses until adulthood and occasionally forever. Characteristically, multiple joints are involved in each patient. Phalangeal, temporomandibular, or vertebral joints have rarely been sites of "spontaneous" hemarthroses within the scope of our experience. The reasons for the high incidence of knee, elbow, and ankle involvements are not clear; however, the lack of protective muscular coverings as well as the shearing forces acting across these joints are undoubtedly major factors. The stress of ordinary daily activities operating on damaged or poorly aligned joints may produce hemorrhage, thus perpetuating a cycle of recurrence.

Apparently, three pathologic processes combine to produce classic hemophilic arthropathy: (1) hemorrhage and the synovial response to it; (2) progressive degeneration of articular cartilage; and (3) the formation of subchondral cysts. Hemorrhage from the synovium and the subsynovial vascular plexus is believed to produce the acute hemarthroses. While a single bleeding episode may produce no significant permanent alteration in the normal joint, multiple bleeding episodes incite an inflammatory response in the hemophilic synovium. Eventually, synovial hyperplasia and hypervascularity result and produce more frequent hemorrhages.[1,2]

Decreased joint mobility results from the coalescence of adjacent villi, the formation of intra-articular fibrous adhesions through incomplete clot resorption, and periarticular fibrosis. Consequently, subtle alterations of the joint biomechanics increase the stress upon the articular complex and render it more susceptible to minor trauma.

Simultaneously, the nutrient function of the synovial membrane is disturbed; cartilage cells disintegrate. The hyaline matrix, deprived of its nutrition and progressively attacked by enzymes released from the inflammatory synovium, softens and wears away.[2] Invasive pannus formation, similar to that of rheumatoid arthritis, occurs and accelerates the degeneration of the articular cartilage.

As the cartilage erodes and its shock absorbing properties are lost, the subchondral bone is subjected to abnormal stress. Microfractures occur; the resultant small intraosseous hemorrhages apparently compromise the circulation within the cancellous bone. The brittle dead bone perpetuates the cycle of microfracture leading to further bone necrosis. As these areas unite, subchondral cysts are formed.[3] Undoubtedly, the encroaching synovium is a factor in producing pressure erosion of the bone; at surgery, larger cysts have been found to be filled with synovial tissue.[4]

A fourth factor should be considered in the pathogenesis of hemophilic arthropathy; the open epiphyses of young patients are involved in the process. Chronic regional hyperemia of the neighboring epiphyseal cartilages, induced by the recurrent hemarthrosis, is believed responsible for the accelerated maturation and hypertrophy of the epiphyseal centers.[5] The growth may be asymmetrical and with partial premature closure of the epiphyses contributes to the angular deformation of the joint and its subsequent early degeneration.

EVALUATION OF ACUTE PROBLEMS

Symptoms of joint stiffness, discomfort, and pain are useful guidelines since they often appear before any swelling is apparent. Proper evaluation of the bleeding episode is paramount and is best accomplished through education of the patient, the parent, and the professional staff. Instruction in hemorrhage assessment includes information about pertinent signs and symptoms of the most common hemorrhages. Special emphasis is given to the types of hemorrhages which are major hazards and to the recognition and the differentiation of soft tissue and joint hemorrhages. Patients, even at a young age, can learn to distinguish changes in their extremities from one day to the next or to recognize unusual bodily occurrences during the day.

A nurse or a physician usually evaluates acute problems in the outpatient transfusion area. It is desirable to have a physical therapist or other musculoskeletal expert available to assess joint and muscle function following acute hemorrhage. Active, not forced, joint motion is measured following hemarthrosis; joints proximal and distal to soft tissue areas are checked when hemorrhage has occurred into calves, thighs, arms, and forearms. Daily circumference measurements, taken at established intervals throughout the extent of the hematoma by the patient or parent, provide some indication of increased or decreased swelling. Daily sensory review is especially important when bleeding has occurred into forearm, popliteal, and iliopsoas areas.

Muscle function is examined following the resolution of an acute joint hemorrhage since muscle weakness occurs rapidly with recurrent joint hemorrhage and predisposes the inadequately supported joint to subsequent hemorrhage. Prompt diagnosis of muscle dysfunction will facilitate the institution of corrective measures to attempt to prevent some future bleeding episodes. Evaluation of muscle function is especially important with transient neuropathy, particularly where finger and thumb functions are impaired. Examination of the involved area is repeated until the hemorrhage has resolved adequately.

THE MANAGEMENT OF ACUTE HEMARTHROSES

Signs and symptoms of joint bleeding include an initial feeling of discomfort or slight stiffness in the affected joint, an increase in local surface temperature, and progressive restriction of joint motion. Varying amounts of swelling and pain depend upon the extent of the hemorrhage, the availability of joint space, and the quickness of hemorrhagic control; muscle "guarding" to immobilize the joint may produce muscle spasm. Ecchymotic areas are usually absent. Patients from an early age can distinguish the presence of joint bleeding before visible, external signs are present. If untreated, bleeding continues until intra-articular pressure exceeds that of the capillaries and the arterioles of the bleeding site.

As elucidated in previous chapters, plasma concentrates and cryoprecipitates are used therapeutically for all suspected hemarthroses and soft tissue hemorrhages. Patients, parents, and the professional staff are encouraged to recognize and treat these bleeding episodes immediately. Ordinarily, *those hemarthroses with minimal pain and minimal to moderate effusion require neither immobilization nor aspiration.* However, arthrocentesis, performed by the resident staff and described in Chapter 4, is attempted when moderate to marked effusion and pain and/or motion restriction are evident in knees, elbows, or ankles (Fig. 6-1). Particularly for the latter two joints, the removal of even small volumes of fluid may produce marked pain relief.

Extremities are immobilized when acute pain or motion restriction is incapacitating. In these cases, plasma products may not have been administered in sufficient dosages or not promptly at the onset of bleeding. When the acute episode is resolved, daytime immobilization is discontinued but nighttime protection may continue for several more days.

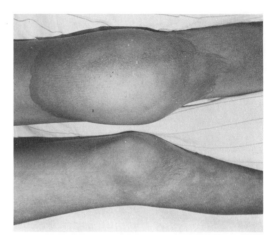

Figure 6-1. A marked hemarthrosis which resulted from delayed concentrate administration and which required arthrocentesis.

Immobilization splints, padded or altered for comfort, are provided for home use by the patient or his parent. The usual precautions are taken to check pressure areas, to ascertain circulatory or sensory impairment, and to determine any adverse effect of the appliance. Some patients adopt the routine application of elastic bandages at the first sign of joint discomfort and credit some lessening of symptomatology to this bandage. The efficacy of this procedure has not been tested; hence, it has neither been encouraged nor discouraged. Many patients utilize cold packs or ice applications for brief periods for the relief of pain of the acute hemorrhage.

Ordinarily, patients are permitted to continue necessary daily activities during acute hemorrhagic episodes depending upon the severity and location of the hemorrhage. Crutches or even a wheelchair may be needed for several days when a severe episode or bilateral problems occur.

Acute and Subacute Knee Hemarthroses

The knee, the most common site of joint bleeding, exhibits varying degrees of swelling usually about suprapatellar or infrapatellar areas; in patients with decreased joint space, only minimal swelling may be discernible. The joint assumes a flexed position with restriction of both extension and flexion; weight bearing is difficult or impossible. Differentiation between a hemorrhage and chronic synovial effusion may not be clear; therefore, bleeding is assumed in these instances. In the hundreds of knee arthrocenteses performed at this Center in the past five years, fewer than five produced a nonsanguineous aspirate.

Considerable attention is directed toward management of the sequelae of bleeding into the knee because of the frequency of these hemorrhages. Early administration of concentrate or cryoprecipitate is essential; immobilization may be necessary for three or four days if pain and/or swelling are marked.

We have employed three types of immobilizing splints including two devices which adjust to the comfortable position of knee extension-flexion:

(1) A molded, thermoplastic splint, with a thigh-to-ankle posterior shell and a lower leg anterior section, is contoured to

the extremity (Fig. 6-2). However, this splint is unsuitable when the acute flexion deformity exceeds 25 to 30 degrees. The splint, attached with Velcro straps, is remoldable as the leg changes in configuration. This appliance is used also to support the leg when walking is resumed after an acute hemorrhage if muscle strength is inadequate to properly protect the knee and is worn until muscular support becomes adequate. This period may be two weeks to several months. Instructions for fabrication and remolding of the device are found in Appendix 3.

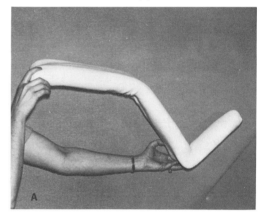

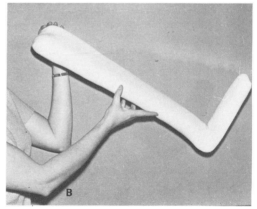

Figure 6-3A and B. Wire frame splint adjusted from flexed to extended position.

(2) When the knee assumes a position of flexion greater than 30 degrees, a padded wire-frame splint is useful (Fig. 6-3). The flexibility of the wire permits daily adjustment of the angle of the knee to allow gradual extension. The device effectively restricts undesirable, premature ambula-

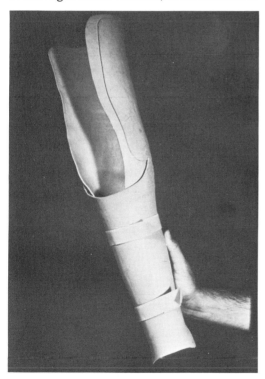

Figure 6-2. Thermoplastic splint.

tion in young patients. The metal frame for this splint can be prepared from flexible wire of ⅜ inch diameter by an orthotic firm or by the engineering services of a hospital. A wooden board, ¼ to ⅜ inches thick and 8 to 10 inches long serves as the foot plate. Cotton padding is wrapped about the wire in a horizontal fashion and covered with tubular stockinette.

(3) A posterior plaster mold immobilizes the knee but new splints are necessary as the joint angle changes. Plaster is inexpensive, universally available, and easily applied; in many situations it is the material of choice. Precautions are necessary to assure sufficient padding over bony prominences and to ensure no pressure or restriction over the bleeding joint.

When the pain factor will permit motion, active exercise begins with concentrate administered prior to the exercise period. Residual quadriceps weakness and loss of knee extension are especially important factors in determining the need for an exercise program. No attempt is made to forcibly extend the knee during the acute/subacute stage. Quadriceps setting and cautious knee extension exercises are begun initially with active ankle and hip motions being instituted at the same time (Figs. 6-4 and 6-5). Patellar mobility is emphasized as shown in Figure 6-6. At any point in the program, when isotonic movements produce pain, isometric exercise can be performed at various positions of the available arc of motion (Fig. 6-7). Trunk flexion and extension exercises are included as well as exercise to all other limbs (Fig. 6-8). Activity in a pool is a valuable adjunct to the dry land regimen.

As the knee passes to the subacute and

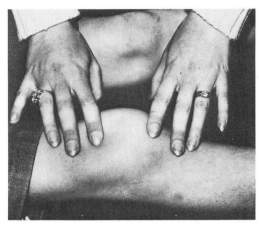

Figure 6-6. Emphasize patellar mobility.

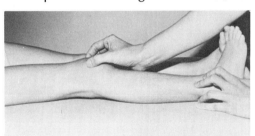

Figure 6-4. Isometric quadriceps exercise.

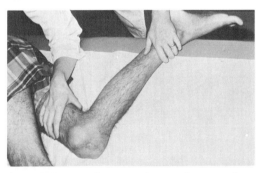

Figure 6-7. Knee flexion and extension at various positions of the motion arc.

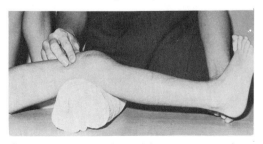

Figure 6-5. Cautious limited knee extension from minimal flexion.

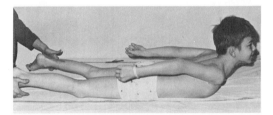

Figure 6-8. Shoulder extension and scapular adduction combined with hip and knee extension.

chronic stages of resolution of the hemorrhages, exercises for the entire involved leg increase in number and intensity. Knee extension from a flexed position may be attempted although patellofemoral pain may be a limiting factor (Fig. 6-9). Rhythmic stabilization and proprioceptive neuromuscular facilitation techniques may be helpful to elicit maximal response (Fig. 6-10). Resistance equipment may be utilized (Figs. 6-11 and 6-12).

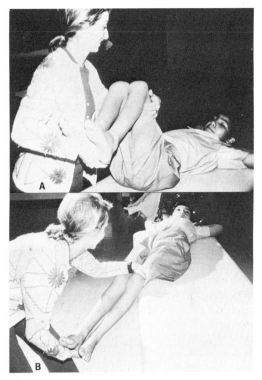

Figure 6-10.

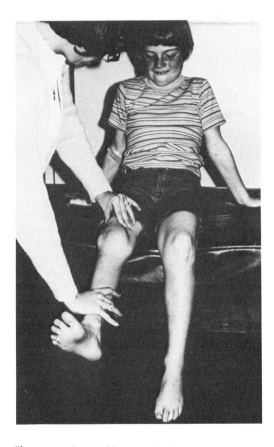

Figure 6-9. Resisted knee extension.

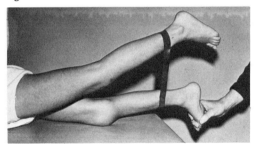

Figure 6-11. Section from tire inner tube for resistance.

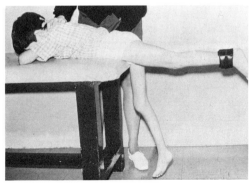

Figure 6-12. Hip extension from flexion with weighted cuff.

Considerable emphasis is placed on strengthening antigravity muscle groups to allow eventual discontinuation of supportive ambulatory devices. However, recent studies by Boone and coworkers indicate that preservation of an arc of knee motion of at least 90 degrees should assume considerable importance when the energy expenditure of walking is evaluated.[6] In selected hemophilic subjects, as the arc of flexion of the most restricted knee decreased below 90 degrees, their oxygen consumption per kg per meter increased. (The selected subjects had restricted knee motion unilateral or bilateral, and motion within normal limits at hips and ankles.)

Weight bearing begins on the involved limb when the *acute* knee flexion deformity approximates the patient's normal position or is less than 25 degrees and the amount of pain or discomfort produced by walking is normal for the patient. As described previously, support of the thermoplastic splint continues until strength of antigravity musculature, especially the quadriceps, is grade good (four) or better and the flexion deformity is 15 degrees or less. Walking distance and endurance increase daily. When antigravity muscle strength has increased to nearly normal, the patient is placed on a maintenance home exercise program which is reviewed and revised periodically by the physical therapist.

The following case history describes the management of recurrent hemarthroses into one knee.

A five-year-old boy, with von Willebrand's disease and less than 1 percent Factor VIII, was referred to the Center because of persistent, repeated hemarthroses into the right knee. For two months prior to evaluation, he was unable to bear weight on the right leg because of hemarthroses and pain; he used a wheelchair for all transportation. Examination revealed a marked effusion of the right knee with 20 degrees loss of complete extension and marked muscle atrophy of thigh and calf groups. Quadriceps strength was assessed at grade

trace (one). Radiographically, mild hemophilic arthritis and joint capsule distention of the right knee were evident.

An intensive, outpatient physical therapy program was instituted to strengthen all muscle groups of the lower extremities and trunk, to improve joint motion where restricted, to encourage device-free ambulation as muscle strength permitted, and to instruct his mother in a comprehensive exercise program as well as details of musculoskeletal management. Prophylactic cryoprecipitate was administered every other day. An opened-thigh thermoplastic splint was fabricated for ambulation and use of the wheelchair was discontinued within the first week of treatment. This program continued for five weeks at which time right knee motion was 0 degrees to 80 degrees and muscle strength of lower extremity groups except the right quadriceps was in the good to normal range (four to five). The right quadriceps was grade fair (three). The patient had learned to swim and to ride a tricycle; he was walking for brief periods each day without the thermoplastic splint. He and his mother returned to their home in South America with complete instructions about progression of the exercise program, evaluation of subsequent hemorrhages, and the use of supportive devices. Correspondence from her indicated that he continued the exercise and physical activity program and within a few weeks was able to discard the thermoplastic splint.

Acute Elbow Hemarthroses

The elbow, subject to the second most commonly occurring hemarthroses, exhibits swelling which is diffuse about the joint or localized at radioulnar, ulnohumeral, or radiohumeral articulations. The joint is maintained in a flexed position with restriction of extension-flexion and pronation-supination. Pain is usually severe and secondarily limits hand, wrist, and shoulder movement.

Following routine administration of concentrate, temporary immobilization is indicated frequently since self-restriction of hand and arm activity is difficult. During the period of resolution, repetitive elbow and forearm motions related to hand and wrist usage, such as typing or prolonged writing, may precipitate a recurrence. Devices to maintain quiescence include:

(1) An inexpensive, readily available cloth sling supports the joint but protects it minimally from external trauma. Shoulder stiffness may occur secondary to prolonged use of the sling.

(2) A posterior plaster shell conforms to the extremity's contours but its rigidity may be difficult for the patient to tolerate.

(3) The most commonly used appliance is an elbow brace, which is adjustable in various attitudes of flexion and extension and which was designed by the author. Use of the hand and shoulder is possible with minimal disturbance of the elbow (Fig. 6-13). This splint is worn for several days following an acute hemorrhage and for two or more weeks during sleep since recurrence of a hemorrhage may be traced to lying on the arm while sleeping or to injuring the elbow on the bed frame. With persistent elbow episodes, patients are encouraged to apply the brace at the first appearance of symptoms and to wear it for several weeks. This elbow brace is constructed of aluminum bars with felt cuffs from the patient's measurements by an orthotist.

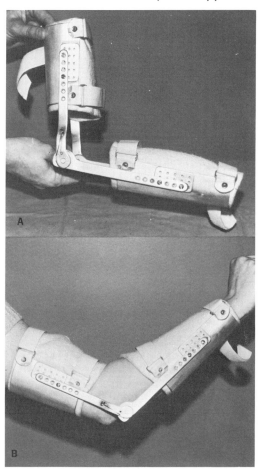

Figure 6-13A and B. Aluminum elbow support with spring-pin mechanism to maintain dial lock in various flexion-extension settings.

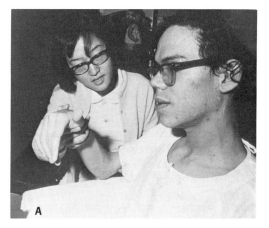

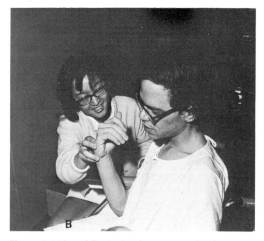

Figure 6-14A and B. Active forearm supination exercise.

When pain-free function is possible, elbow and forearm active motion begins; the patient may continue to wear the splint, but removes it for daily exercise periods. Markedly improved joint motion rarely occurs with exercise once chronic restriction is evident; therefore, exercise is directed toward muscle strengthening within the existing arcs of motion. Pronation and supination are emphasized since these rotary forearm movements are more essential in daily activity than the extreme limits of flexion and extension (Fig. 6-14). Passive stretching or forced elbow motion are not indicated. Shoulder, wrist, and hand exercises are included.

Acute Ankle Hemarthroses

The ankle presents swelling of varying amounts about the talofibular or talotibial articulations. Extension, flexion, and forefoot motions are limited with the ankle maintained in slight flexion. Severe pain is usual and prohibits functional weight bearing.

The majority of ankle episodes require neither splinting nor arthrocentesis; however, a posterior plaster splint immobilizes those hemarthroses which exhibit effusion and marked pain. The splint is used until ambulation is resumed at which time the canvas anklet, described below, is applied.

When the pain factor becomes negligible, talar and subtalar motions are begun. Attention is directed to increasing ankle extension (dorsiflexion) and flexion (plantar flexion); however, use of toe extensors to attempt to extend the ankle is discouraged. Hammertoe deformities can result from this practice; better balanced muscle power and stimulation of tibialis anterior action may reduce the occurrence of these deformities. Instruction in and practice of a proper heel-to-toe gait pattern is important.

Supportive footwear, such as Italian hiking boots, desert boots, or high top tennis shoes, is indicated for patients incurring occasional ankle hemarthroses. When hemarthroses are frequent, additional support is provided by a laced canvas anklet, with medial and lateral metal stays, which is accommodated by regular footwear (Fig. 6-15). Its use is gradually discontinued as the condition of the ankle stabilizes; however, during periods of recreational exercise, such as tennis, the patient may elect to wear the support as a protective measure. This support is supplied to orthotists by Tru-Form Anatomical Supports, Cincinnati, Ohio 45209.

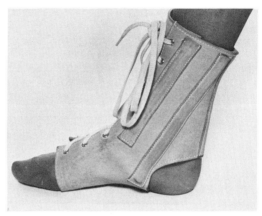

Figure 6-15. Laced canvas anklet.

Hip Hemarthroses

With severe hemorrhage into the hip, acute distention may be palpable; the joint assumes a flexed position and protects against rotational or abducted movements. All planes of movement are markedly restricted; attempted motion produces severe pain. Differentiation between hip hemorrhage and iliopsoas bleeding may be puzzling. Two tests are usually discriminatory:

(1) When the patient flexes the trunk (performs a sit-up), severe pain is produced in the presence of iliopsoas bleeding while only mild or absent pain is found with a hip hemorrhage.

(2) When the examiner gently rotates the flexed hip inwardly and outwardly, severe pain is evident with the hip hemorrhage and is mild or absent when there is iliopsoas bleeding.

Hospitalization is often necessary for management of this major hemorrhage with dosage of the plasma products adjusted accordingly. Traction may produce pain relief during the acute and subacute period; oral steroids may reduce the characteristic synovitis. (Refer to Chap. 3). Occasionally, a severe hemorrhage responds to aspiration but this is undertaken with great caution and only when more conservative measures have failed to provide relief. Following resolution of the episode and reduction of pain, exercise focuses on hip extension and abduction within the pain-free arcs of motion; exercise is initiated in the water prior to a dry land program. Strengthening exercises are included for the thigh and the lower leg musculature as well as for the contralateral extremity. The use of crutches or canes may be necessary for varying periods of time depending upon the extent and frequency of the hemorrhages; however, continuous use of these devices may precipitate elbow and shoulder hemarthroses in the younger patient.

Young patients with recurrent hemorrhages are encouraged to remain as physically active as possible during the intervals when they are without acute or subacute symptoms, even when mild to moderate degenerative changes are present. However, jumping and running activities are discouraged. The importance of dietary control is emphasized at an early age since obesity will increase the stress on the diseased hip. Complete confinement to the bed or to the wheelchair was routine treatment until eight years ago. However, immobility did not appear to alter the degenerative process, created positional restriction of other joints, and produced negative behavioral reactions in the patient.

Shoulder and Wrist Hemarthroses

With shoulder hemarthroses, acute distention may be palpable and the joint may assume a dependent, adducted position with resistance to attempted passive movements. All planes of motion, especially flexion, abduction, and rotation, are markedly reduced. Marked pain is present.

In addition to the infusion of plasma products, support of the extremity in a sling may reduce the discomfort of an acute hemorrhage for some patients; others obtain relief through gravitational traction. Subsequent exercises are directed toward improving joint motion in all planes but especially flexion, abduction, and rotation. Proprioceptive neuromuscular facilitation patterns and rhythmic stabilization techniques are used to advantage with shoulder and upper extremity involvement. Certain swimming strokes, particularly the back stroke and the crawl or modifications of them, are beneficial when more vigorous activity can be undertaken.

Wrist hemarthroses are infrequent but should be differentiated from volar soft tissue hemorrhage.

HEMORRHAGE INTO THE SOFT TISSUE OF THE EXTREMITIES

Bleeding may occur in any body area, however, flexor surfaces appear to have a higher incidence than extensor surfaces of extremities. Sizable volumes of blood can be lost into thighs, calves, forearms, and retroperitoneal cavities. Vascular compression may lead to localized ischemia and necrosis while neural compression will result in transient or occasionally persistent motor and sensory deficits. Fibrous tissue may replace muscle fibers and may produce secondary contracture of adjacent joints. Recurrence of hemorrhage is common particularly in the lower extremity.

Signs and symptoms of significant soft tissue hemorrhage include an initial feeling of discomfort or pain which progresses in intensity, motion restriction of those joints associated with the muscle groups involved in the hemorrhage, and swelling or distention palpable by careful examination. Ecchymotic areas are not usually evident with the acute hemorrhage but eventual discoloration may occur. As the hemorrhage progresses, skin areas become glossy in appearance; extensive swelling and increased local temperature are found. Areas of numbness or tingling may be present.

Bleeding into certain areas presents challenges to treatment because of the potential for development of long standing deformity.

Hemorrhage into the Gastrocnemius-Soleus Calf Group

The hemorrhage may be located anywhere from the origins of the gastrocnemius-soleus muscles to their insertion. Marked distention of the entire calf is common with the knee and the ankle assuming positions of flexion.

Protection of the calf area is provided by the flexible, padded wire splint previously described. The splint, comfortably positioned to exert no tension on the calf, popliteal, or posterior thigh areas and adjusted to accommodate increased knee and ankle extension, is worn until ambulation is safely resumed. Methods such as traction or forcibly attempted knee extension are contraindicated because they precipitate rebleeding. Walking may begin when the entire foot is in contact with the floor with the knee in a position of less than 20 degrees flexion or the leg has returned to its prehemorrhagic status. The period of recuperation may be several weeks for a severe hemorrhage; plasma products are administered for several days to several weeks during this period dependent upon the severity of the episode. Occasionally, ultrasound has been empirically administered to hasten absorption of the hematoma. Recurrence of hemorrhage is frequent when walking is attempted in the face of moderate ankle and knee flexion deformity. Additionally, the stresses placed upon the knee joint in this mechanically-poor position may precipitate a knee hemarthrosis, further complicating the recovery period.

Gentle active knee and ankle exercise emphasizing extension is instituted when the swelling and the local temperature have decreased and the pain is minimal. Again, common toe extensors should not be used alone to attempt to produce ankle extension. A persistent knee flexion deformity is managed as described in the section on chronic knee problems. When

hemorrhages into the calf group muscles are treated adequately and soon after their occurrence, persistant residual deformity is not evident.

The potential for permanent deformity following inadequate treatment of a severe hemorrhage into the calf is illustrated by the following case history:

An 11-year-old boy with severe hemophilia A (less than 1 percent Factor VIII) was examined one year following a severe hemorrhage into the left calf which had been treated in his community hospital with bedrest and minimal, infrequent dosages of fresh-frozen plasma. A 45 degree loss of knee extension and a 35 degree equinus deformity were present as seen in Figure 6-16. He

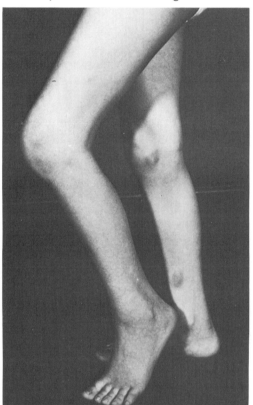

Figure 6-16.

had been essentially nonambulatory for the year following the original hemorrhage. Because his referral to the Center preceded the commercial availability of plasma concentrate or cryoprecipitate, surgical correction of the deformities was not possible. He was hospitalized for corrective casting and intensive exercise for a six week period. Exercise was performed in and out of water to attempt to improve knee and ankle motion and to strengthen major muscle groups of the lower extremities and the trunk. Opened-thigh cylinder casts, bivalved for removal during exercise, were utilized for a six month period to maintain the corrected positions of knee and ankle extension. At that time, extension-flexion of the left knee was 10 to 100 degrees and the equinus position of the ankle was reduced to 5 degrees, as shown in Figure 6-17. He was seen on a regular, monthly

basis as an outpatient for the next three years and less frequently for the subsequent seven years. At the time of his last examination, ten years from his initial contact with us, he had maintained knee motion of 10 to 125 degrees; the equinus position persisted at 10 degrees. He has incurred periodic hemarthroses into the left knee with resultant degenerative changes; these hemorrhages have been managed at home by self-infusion of plasma concentrate or cryoprecipitate. The residual plantar flexion deformity and the knee arthropathy may produce functional problems for him at a later date.

Iliopsoas Hemorrhage

Iliopsoas hemorrhage is potentially life threatening due to the severe blood loss since bleeding can dissect through tissues into adjacent areas and thus produce a sizable, diffuse hematoma. The exact location of the hemorrhage is often evasive; however, the sheath of the iliacus muscle has been reported to be the site of the bleeding with secondary distention into the psoas area.[7] Pain, localizing in the groin or lower quadrant area, is usually extreme. The leg on the involved side assumes a hip-flexed position (Fig. 6-18). A

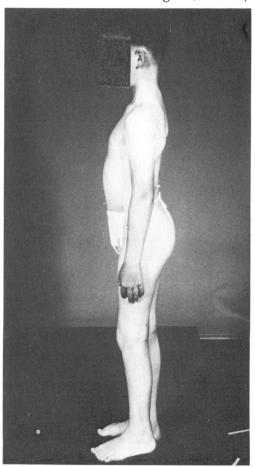

Figure 6-17.

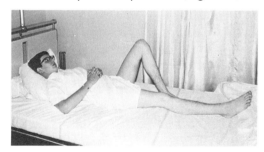

Figure 6-18. Left iliopsoas hemorrhage with characteristic hip-flexed position.

mass can usually be palpated in the iliac fossa although it may not be evident for two to three days from onset. Differentiation from appendicitis and hip hemarthrosis is essential. (Refer to discriminatory tests in the section on hip hemarthrosis in this chapter.) Femoral nerve compression will produce transient sensory and motor deficits. In spite of hospitalization and massive doses of plasma concentrates, recurrence is frequent and often coincides with the resumption of ambulation. The greatest apparent incidence occurs in patients from their early teens to their mid-twenties.

The involved limb is maintained in a position of comfort, which is usually with neutral hip rotation and considerable flexion. No attempt is made to forcibly increase hip extension; the application of *traction* is *contraindicated* because a recurrence of hemorrhage and additional pain ordinarily results from its use. With a severe hemorrhage, concentrate infusion, analgesic administration and bedrest may be the only course of management for several days.

Electrical stimulation precedes active exercise when paresis is evident in the quadriceps muscle group. Exercise is not begun to any part of the body until the extreme pain in the groin, flank, or hip area has subsided and the position of hip flexion is 45 degrees or less. Additionally, the patient must be able to move from his bed to a stretcher or wheelchair with minimal difficulty and without a perceptible increase in pain. Exercise is begun in a pool with *minimal movement* of the involved extremity for two or three days. The uninvolved limbs are used to move about in the water. After the few days, gentle, active motions of hip, knee, and ankle of the symptomatic leg begin; exercise is suspended if any increased pain or discomfort occurs in the groin or hip area.

Walking is not permitted until the hip flexion position is 25 degrees or less; when instituted with the hip in more flexion, rehemorrhage is common. Crutch support is usual until the flexion deformity is further reduced to 10 to 15 degrees. When quadriceps weakness or paresis is present, the anterior opened-thigh cylinder cast is utilized to support the knee. The support is maintained until the strength of the quadriceps and other antigravity muscles is at least grade good. With severe motor and sensory impairment, the return to the functional pre-

hemorrhagic state may require six or more months. The following case histories delineate management of severe hemorrhages in a patient with an inhibitor and in a patient with mild hemophilia. The first case was without neurologic deficit.

A 20-year-old man with less than 1 percent Factor VIII and a circulating inhibitor was hospitalized with a diagnosis of left iliopsoas hemorrhage. His left hip was positioned in 90 degrees of flexion; he complained of severe pain in the left groin and lower quadrant area. No neurologic impairment was evident. He was placed on bedrest with adequate analgesia; 10 mg of prednisolone was administered three times per day for four days, and 5 mg three times per day for the following 20 days. An initial attempt was made to administer a massive dosage of Factor VIII concentrate to achieve a satisfactory plasma level; however, this attempt was unsuccessful and further infusions were not attempted. Exercise began in the pool approximately two and one-half weeks after admission when the hip flexion position had decreased to 45 degrees. He began ambulating on crutches for very limited periods four weeks after admission; his active exercise program continued. At discharge, after six weeks' hospitalization he was using crutches and his hip position was reduced to 30 degrees flexion. He was seen on a regular outpatient basis for six months at which time no residual of the hemorrhage was evident. Subsequent examinations revealed no recurrence of the problem; normal motions of the left hip, knee, and ankle were evident 18 months and 3 years later. Muscular development was within normal limits.

The second case illustrates recurrence of hemorrhage with motor and sensory involvement.

An 18-year-old boy with 11 percent Factor VIII presented with his fourth iliopsoas hemorrhage in three years. All four episodes were precipitated by participation in competitive athletic endeavors or the physical conditioning required prior to participation. Although Center personnel discouraged his involvement in track and field activities following the initial iliopsoas hemorrhage, he persisted in active competition in high school athletic events and had been offered a college scholarship because of his abilities. He was without neuromuscular sequela from the previous bleeding episodes prior to this right iliopsoas hemorrhage for which he was hospitalized for 27 days. At the time of hospital admission, extreme pain and tenderness were present throughout his right groin and lower abdominal area; his right hip was in 75 degrees flexion. Motor and sensory losses were complete for the femoral nerve distribution.

Treatment for a two week period consisted of twice daily infusion of cryoprecipitate (to maintain Factor VIII levels of 50 percent), bedrest in the position of comfort, adequate analgesia, and galvanic stimulation to the quadriceps muscle group. Active exercise of the left leg, arms, and trunk began in the pool two weeks after hospital admission at which time the hip was in a position of 35 degrees flexion. His program gradually progressed to include active exercise for the right hip, knee, and ankle and protected walking. At the time of discharge, he was ambulatory with crutches and a thermoplastic splint. Some areas of hypersensitivity as well as hypoesthesia were found on the anterior and lateral thigh; quadriceps strength was grade poor (two). He continued the exercise program as an outpatient. At the time of his last follow-up appointment, three months after the episode, sensory impairment was still evident throughout the anterior right thigh; quadriceps strength was grade fair (three).

Forearm Hematoma

Forearm hemorrhage is common in the volar wrist area but may be situated anywhere between the wrist and elbow. A volar hematoma may compress ulnar or median nerve branches producing motor and sensory deficits of the palm, the thumb, and/or the fingers. The hematoma may extend into the palmar aponeurosis and the flexor sheaths. Usually, the wrist assumes a flexed position with the fingers held in varying amounts of flexion. Active finger motions of extension, flexion, abduction, and adduction are impaired as are thumb opposition, flexion, and abduction. Pain is usual and may be accompanied by tingling, itching sensations, or varying degrees of numbness.

In the initial posthemorrhagic period, splinting the hand and wrist may be impossible due to severe pain. As the pain subsides, a well padded volar splint, fabricated of thermoplastic material or plaster, is molded to maintain the hand and wrist in a more functional posture. As the hemorrhage resolves, the splint is realigned with the hand and wrist. As active wrist, finger, and thumb functions return, the splint is discontinued. Electrical stimulation of intrinsic and extrinsic hand musculature is indicated when marked motor deficits are found. Active hand and finger exercise emphasizing grasp and oppositional activities, are encouraged as the hematoma resolves. With early treatment and prompt, correct evaluation of the problem, complete recovery without functional deficits is usual; however, with delayed or inadequate treatment, horrendous deformities and complete loss of function of the hand and fingers are frequent occurrences.

The following case histories illustrate the effectiveness of early management and the dire consequences of neglect:

A 10-year-old boy with severe hemophilia A (less than 1 percent factor VIII) was seen in the outpatient treatment area with a severe hemorrhage into the volar aspect of the left wrist extending into the palmar surface of the hand; the hemorrhage was of several hours' duration (Fig. 6-19). Pain and numbness were evident in the cutaneous distribution of the median nerve.

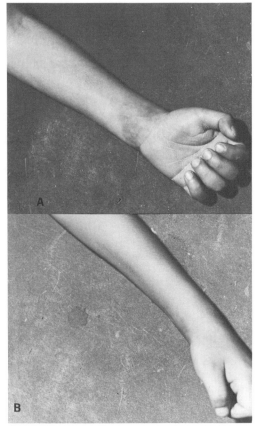

Figure 6-19A and B. Position of fingers, thumb, and wrist at time of initial examination.

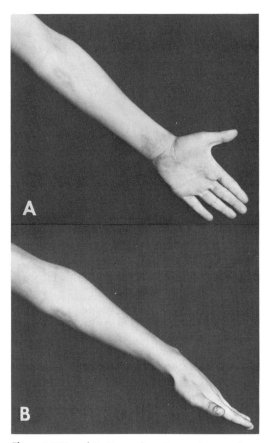

Figure 6-20A and B. Normal motion and motor function.

Thenar motor activity was absent; circulation was intact. Because of transportation difficulties and poor follow-up of instructions at home, hospitalization was deemed essential for a five day period. During this period, Factor VIII concentrate was administered daily; a volar plaster splint was fabricated. At the time of discharge, hypoesthesia was limited to the immediate median nerve distribution; thenar motor activity was detectable but quite weak. He was followed every other day for two weeks as an outpatient for administration of concentrate and evaluation of the status of the hand. Active exercise of the thumb and fingers was encouraged as muscle activity was reestablished. Two months following the initial hemorrhage, median hypoesthesia persisted in the thumb and a portion of the index

finger; no residual loss of motion of fingers or thumb was evident and motor function was nearly normal (Fig. 6-20).

This result is in direct contrast to that of the following patient:

This 28-year-old man was referred to the Center for evaluation and treatment of a right Volkmann's ischemic contracture which had reportedly existed for three months prior to examination. A history of a massive forearm hemorrhage secondary to trauma was elicited. *In spite of his known diagnosis of severe hemophilia (less than 1 percent Factor VIII) he had received no treatment for the hemorrhage in his home community.* Evaluation revealed only 30 degrees motion present in his elbow with no supination or pronation capability; the wrist was fixed in marked flexion. Motion of his proximal phalanges was approximately 20 degrees; none was present in the distal phalanges. Motor and sensory impairment of the ulnar and median nerve distributions was evident. Although this had been his dominant extremity, he was unable to use it for any daily functions. Surgical intervention, instituted to at tempt to improve the position of the hand and the wrist and to provide some useful finger function, included neurolysis of the ulnar and median nerves, excision of the necrotic portions of the flexor digitorum profundus and the flexor carpi radialis, transfer of the flexor digitorum sublimis to the profundus tendons and the transfer of the palmaris longus to the flexor pollicis longus. Recovery was complicated by the formation of an abscess in the volar aspect of the wrist. Hematologic management became difficult as well when the patient developed a low level inhibitor to Factor VIII several days following surgery. He was hospitalized for a period of two months. Six months after discharge no useful function of the arm distal to the elbow was evident; the severe sensory disturbance persisted. Minimal tenodesis action of the finger flexors was present secondary to wrist extension. He was unable to return to his previous vocation and was considered a poor candidate for retraining because of his multiple physical disabilities and his limited education.

Other Soft Tissue Hemorrhages

Hemorrhage into the anterior tibial compartment is infrequent but the function of the tibialis anterior and extensor hallucis longus may be temporarily impaired. This hemorrhage results commonly from the pressure of a cylinder cast. Signs of lower leg numbness or inactivity of the noted muscles should be anticipated when a cast is present. Prevention of an equinus deformity is essential to provide a mechanically sound weight bearing posture in the future. A lightweight spring brace, often required when walking is resumed, is used until the anterior lower leg musculature is sufficiently strong to extend the foot and toes for clearance of the foot during walking.

Posterior thigh hemorrhage is usually the result of trauma which may be as simple as sitting with considerable impact on a noncushioned chair or stool. Management is essentially as described under gastrocnemius-soleus hemorrhage but compression of the sciatic nerve or its branches is carefully evaluated. A nonrigid support, such as provided by the flexible, padded, wire splint may be used within pain tolerance. Exercise is cautiously instituted as the hematoma resolves with emphasis placed on extensor capacity of the knee and ankle. Weight bearing on the affected limb is not attempted until the knee flexion deformity is less than 25 degrees and the patient's active attempts to extend the knee do not produce pain. Depending upon the presence of neuropathy, the foot and ankle may require support when the patient is upright.

Anterior or lateral thigh, buttock, or upper arm hemorrhages are not as potentially crippling as those just discussed (Fig. 6-21). Motion restriction is transient; ordinarily, mobilization is not difficult after resolution of the hemorrhage.

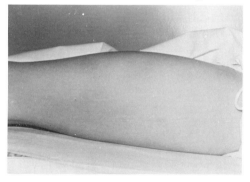

Figure 6-21. Anterolateral thigh hematoma without crippling residual.

EVALUATION OF CHRONIC PROBLEMS

A periodically scheduled musculoskeletal evaluation is valuable for long-term follow-up of these patients. Patterns of the disease process can be identified, decreases of function revealed, and the effectiveness of certain treatment methods evaluated. A brief history is taken to summarize previous bleeding episodes into the extremities, particularly the joints, and to include management of prior musculoskeletal problems. Range of joint motion measurements of shoulders, elbows, wrists, hips, knees, and ankles are obtained initially and repeated at 12 to 18 month intervals. Measurements are taken when the patient is free from acute bleedings. A suggested system of measurement is that of the American Academy of Orthopaedic Surgeons; however, the system of measurement and the testing personnel should be consistent.[8]

Functional information, obtained through observation and interview, includes gait analysis, walking endurance, stair climbing ability, as well as determination of any daily physical obstacles encountered by the patient when he is functioning at his normal level. A notation is made of his type of gait as well as any gross walking abnormalities. Leg lengths are examined supine and standing and a clinical scoliosis examination is performed. The use of or need for assistive devices such as splints, braces, crutches, canes, or wheelchairs is ascertained.

When joint dysfunction and secondary muscle atrophy are apparent, a gross determination of muscle strength is indicated. A more finite examination is indicated when neuropathic residuals are evident. Again, consistency of personnel is important for comparison of one evaluation with subsequent evaluations.

MANAGEMENT OF CHRONIC MUSCULOSKELETAL PROBLEMS

As previously discussed, the musculoskeletal residuals of hemorrhage present the greatest morbidity problems of this disease. Clinically, the repeated hemarthroses and subsequent joint deterioration produce loss of range of joint motion and stiffness coupled with secondary weakness of the muscles associated with that joint. Little correlation is found between the motion and function of the joint and its radiographic appearance. Inequality of leg and arm lengths are common. Morning stiffness and positional gelling, although common, are usually alleviated by activity and are generally present for shorter periods than those experienced by patients with rheumatoid arthritis. Amounts of pain and discomfort vary according to the functional demands placed upon the joint, the environmental conditions, and the patient's tolerance. As the degeneration proceeds and the patient ages, he experiences increasing difficulty in walking, in climbing stairs, and in general mobility. However, in spite of marked degeneration in multiple joints, most adults with severe hemophilia continue to function comparatively well in daily life.

A study of joint motion revealed statistically significant differences between a group of 152 hemophilic and a group of 120 normal male subjects in all motions of the major joints of the body.[9] Measurements of the hemophilic group were conducted prior to the availability of plasma concentrates. When the groups were analyzed by age, the oldest hemophilic subjects exhibited a greater motion loss than did the oldest normal subjects when compared with their youngest counterparts. Surprisingly, even the youngest hemophilic subjects, aged one to five years, evidenced motion deficits when compared with their normal counterparts. Measurements of 105 hemophilics of the study group were repeated nine years later. Data from this subsequent evaluation are currently being analyzed.

Chronic problems of motion restriction, stiffness, discomfort, and residual muscle atrophy are treated initially with exercise. Response to this conservative approach is quite rewarding since the daily function of many patients can be improved even though the chronic joint pathology is unchanged. When more aggressive measures are required, supportive or corrective devices may be used; exercise continues within the limits imposed by the device. When initiating exercises or increasing the intensity of the regimen, plasma products are administered prophylactically prior to exercise to prevent episodes of minor bleeding which will limit the program. Plasma factor levels of 20 to 25 percent are attained for this purpose on a daily basis until the patient and his joints are acclimated to exercise, i.e., muscular support has improved, joint pain or discomfort during exercise has ceased. Exercises can be performed without prior concentrate administration; however, progression from simple to more strenuous resistive exercise will be slower.

Weight control is vitally important for those patients with degenerative hip, knee, and ankle symptomatology since relatively small weight gains are reflected in increased discomfort and in decreased general mobility. Certain analgesic and/or anti-inflammatory medications, discussed in Chapters 2 and 3, may be useful to reduce the arthritic manifestations of recurrent hemarthroses. Warm baths and showers in the morning may be helpful to relieve the stiffness found upon arising. Patients are counseled to keep arthritic joints warm during periods of cold or inclement weather; elastic bandages or commercially available "knee warmers" are useful. Additionally, sitting for prolonged periods of time is discouraged while studying or working, since this position will encourage stiffness. Patients should be made aware of the arthritic nature of many of their complaints so they can attempt to distinguish between the symptoms of a hemarthrosis and those of joint degeneration. The patient should understand that he has a type of arthritis and complete pain relief may be impossible.

Severe degenerative changes in multiple joints accompanied by severe muscle atrophy and prolonged previous disability may present obstacles to functional rehabilitation which are difficult and often impossible to overcome. Particularly in these cases, treatment goals should be clearly defined, understood, and accepted by all members of the treatment team, especially the patient. Often, the realistic goal is less than the ideal rehabilitation goal; recognition and acceptance of these divergencies are essential.

Chronic Knee Involvement

The course of knee involvement in hemophilia has been described frequently as beginning with the repetitive cycle of hemorrhage in childhood and producing a chronic synovitis and a mechanical alteration of joint function.[2] Unless vigorously treated, severe degenerative changes will result by the time of epiphyseal closure. Flexion deformities of varying amounts are often coupled with posterior subluxation of the tibia, increased valgus or varus, and abnormal tibial torsion. Bony overgrowth of the femoral condyles, especially the medial, is a consistent finding (Fig. 6-22). The

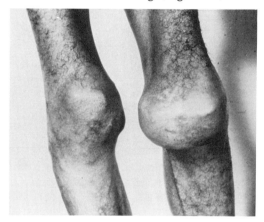

Figure 6-22. Marked overgrowth and angulation deformity of knee of 50-year-old man.

patellofemoral joint is almost always involved to a painful, marked degree that limits the attempts to rehabilitate the thigh musculature, especially the quadriceps group. After skeletal maturity, the limitation of flexion and extension, patellar fixation, and muscular weakness become predominant findings. Management focuses on positioning the knee in a better mechanical attitude for ambulation.

When the knee evidences chronic arthritis and/or synovitis, loss of 15 to 20 degrees complete extension, and atrophy of thigh musculature, an anterior opened-thigh cylinder cast or thermoplastic splint is applied (Fig. 6-23). The materials used in

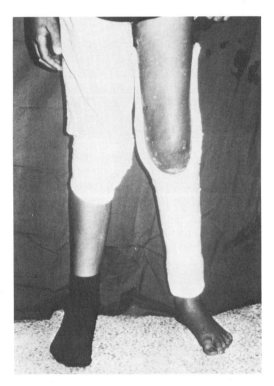

Figure 6-23. Opened-thigh cylinder cast.

the construction depend upon the patient's size and weight, the degree of flexion deformity, and the extent of muscle weakness. The cylinder extends from the gluteal fold to one inch above the malleoli; the anterior thigh portion is removed to the level of the proximal tibial plateau. The anterior lower leg portion may or may not be removable depending upon the condition of the patient's extremity. Ankle and hip function during walking are relatively unrestricted in this support and knee motion of 5 to 10 degrees occurs during ambulation. Vigorous exercise continues during the period when this support is being utilized; emphasis is placed on knee extension activity as well as that of other antigravity musculature.

As muscle atrophy and synovitis decrease, increased extension of the knee usually occurs, although it may be a slow process depending upon the duration of the chronic symptoms. The splint is changed to accompany the new configuration of the knee and thigh (Fig. 6-24). When the flexion deformity has decreased to approximately 10 degrees and quadriceps strength is grade fair (three) or better, the splint is gradually discontinued. If the open-thigh splint was fabricated from plaster, the lower leg portion is bivalved at this time and straps are added for gradual reduction of wearing, or the thermoplastic splint may be substituted. Increased stresses are placed upon the lower extremities through the use of manual resistance, resisted walking exercises, the use of the treadmill, as well as through weights and pulleys (Fig. 6-25). Pool exercise is used to facilitate knee remobilization.

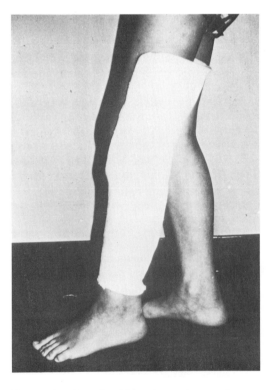

Figure 6-24. Cast should be changed to conform to increased knee extension.

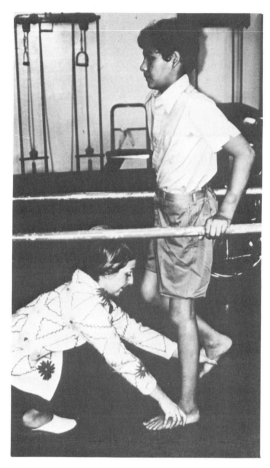

Figure 6-25. Resisted walking following correction of 60 degrees knee flexion deformity.

The following case history illustrates conservative correction of bilateral knee flexion deformities complicated by recurrent fracture of the right tibia:

When this 12-year-old boy with severe Factor VIII deficiency was initially examined, he exhibited knee motion of 30 to 120 degrees on the left and 35 to 140 degrees on the right with secondary bilateral hip flexion deformity of 25 degrees. He had utilized a wheelchair for all transportation for nearly four years. Since his home was over 100 miles from the Center, hospitalizations were necessary during the period of deformity correction which was prolonged because of the fractures. Plasma con-

centrates were unavailable at the time. On radiographs, moderately severe degenerative arthritic changes of the knees (Fig. 6-26), slightly greater on the right, were apparent at the initial contact as were mild changes of both ankles. Exercise and opened-thigh casts were used extensively for an 11 month period at which time motion in the left knee became within normal limits; the right knee progressed more slowly, evidencing only a 15 degree maintained change in extension during the same period. The extension desubluxation hinges, described later in this chapter, did not exist at the time. However, their

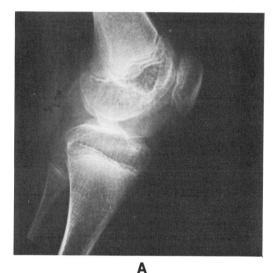

A

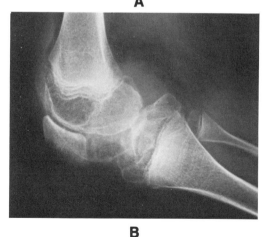

B

Figure 6-26. Initial radiographs of (A) left and (B) right knees.

use would have probably shortened the time required to correct the knee flexion deformities. Two right tibial fractures occurred within the next six months, necessitating immobilization of the right knee and loss of motion. Repeated applications of the opened-thigh cast were required to improve the weight bearing position of the knee when walking resumed; exercise was intensified as well. Three years after the initial evaluation, the right knee had motion of 10 to 95 degrees while the left knee and both hips reflected normal function. Slight motion limitations were found in both ankles. His limbs were essentially the same when he was last examined at age 21 which was nine years from our first contact with him.

Radiographically, moderate degenerative changes were evident in both knees and the right ankle. The hips were normal in appearance. His walking was unrestricted in both distance and terrain. Occasional discomfort in one or both ankles was relieved by the canvas and metal ankle support. He swam, played tennis, softball, and neighborhood basketball and continued to use a stationary bicycle for exercise. He has participated in the home transfusion program since 1968. Psychosocial information about him appears in Chapter 11 identified as Kenny G.

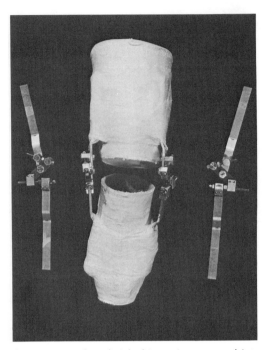

Figure 6-28. Left and right hinges incorporated into plaster cylinders. In actual application, the anterior distal thigh portion should extend over the distal quadriceps-patellar area.

Chronic problems of severe joint restriction, muscle atrophy, tibial subluxation, and moderate to severe degenerative changes require more aggressive methods to extend the knee and to attempt to desubluxate the tibia (Fig. 6-27). A pair of metal extension desubluxation hinges is incorporated into thigh and lower leg plaster cylinders. The foot and ankle are not included in the plaster nor is the area about the knee covered. The hinges with adjustment screws for extension and desubluxation are placed medially and laterally to the knee with the axes of the hinges aligned with the joint line of the knee (Fig. 6-28). Constant corrective forces are applied in gradual daily increments by the patient or his parent following instruction in this procedure. Several times during the day, the patient releases the tension on the extension screws and allows the knee to flex; corrective force is then resumed. The usual precautions are taken to prevent neurovascular impairment or skin prob-

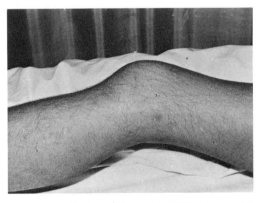

Figure 6-27. Flexion deformity requiring aggressive correction.

lems. A detailed method of application of this corrective appliance is illustrated in Appendix 4. Ordinarily, plasma concentrate is administered to attain prophylactic levels prior to the application of the hinges; during the period of correction, concentrate is administered therapeutically for reported hemorrhages but is not given prophylactically.

Ambulation occurs in the cast with or without crutches. Exercise of the other extremities and the trunk continues as necessary. The patient is instructed to perform isometric knee extension and flexion exercises for the casted extremity as well as active hip and ankle movements. Maximum effectiveness of the extension desubluxation hinges is achieved within a two to three week period. Correction beyond 10 to 15 degrees flexion is not expected; at that point, a cylinder plaster cast replaces the hinged cast and is used to retain the corrected position. The anterior thigh portion is removed in two weeks. The cast in turn is replaced by the thermoplastic splint when quadriceps strength has increased. Serial use of the hinged cast is indicated when attempting to correct flexion deformities greater than 50 degrees.

Ordinarily, the amount of knee flexion does not change through the use of this device; for example, a knee with extension-flexion of 35 to 85 degrees will be corrected to an arc of 15 to 65 degrees. Subsequent increased motion may or may not occur depending upon the extent of the degenerative joint changes, the degree of intra-articular and periarticular fibrosis, and the age of the patient. Often, children will increase knee motion to normal limits following correction of the knee flexion deformity.

G. Carlton Wallace, M.D., designed these extension desubluxation hinges during his resident training period at Orthopaedic Hospital. Modifications of the design were made by William A. Craig, M.D., to reduce the weight of the hinges, originally made from stainless steel, and to eliminate shearing forces on the screws. California Design and Manufacturing Company, 1732 Tanen Street, Napa, California 94558, is the manufacturer and supplier.

The following case histories demonstrate the use of the extension desubluxation hinges to correct short-term as well as long-standing deformity:

A 15-year-old boy (less than 1 percent Factor VIII) was seen with a flexion deformity of the left knee secondary to a hemarthrosis into a knee with existing severe arthropathy. His history included multiple, recurrent bleeding episodes into the left knee since the age of two years. At the time of examination, a flexion deformity of 35 degrees was evident and strength of the quadriceps muscle group was poor. Knee joint motion two months prior to the examination had been 10 to 75 degrees. The increased deformity resisted correction by exercise alone; therefore, an extension desubluxation hinge cast was applied for eight days (Figs. 6-29 and 6-30). When the deformity had been reduced to 10 degrees,

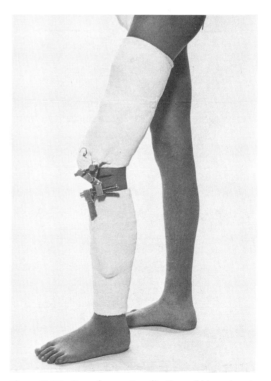

Figure 6-29. One day postapplication of hinged cast. Knee in 30 degrees flexed position.

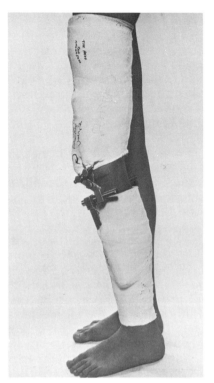

Figure 6-30. On eighth postapplication day with knee in 10 degrees flexion, prior to cast removal.

the hinge cast was removed and an anterior opened-thigh cylinder cast was applied for a 17 day period and then replaced by a thermoplastic splint. A vigorous exercise program preceded by plasma concentrate was implemented during the period of all casting. Six months after the hinge casting, the knee had motion of 10 to 65 degrees; quadriceps strength was fair and the thermoplastic splint was gradually discontinued.

The second case demonstrates correction of long existing deformity prior to the availability of plasma concentrate.

A five-year-old patient, with less than 1 percent Factor IX, was seen with a marked flexion deformity of the left knee which had existed for a two year period and which confined him to a wheelchair. Left knee motion was 95 to 105 degrees; a secondary hip flexion

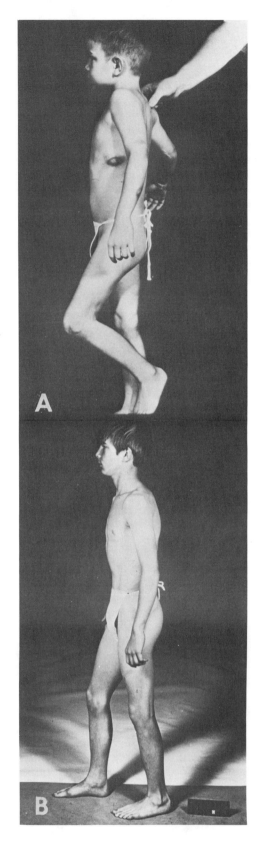

Figure 6-31. A, Patient at initial examination and B, ▶ eight years later.

deformity of 25 degrees was present. During the period of deformity correction, Factor IX concentrate was not manufactured so several months' hospitalization was necessary. Availability of this concentrate would have decreased or eliminated the need for hospitalization and would have reduced greatly the period of time required to obtain correction. Lyophilized plasma was infused to treat any bleeding episodes which occurred during the correction period. Extension desubluxation hinges were applied followed by opened-thigh casts. A four month period was required to obtain a position of only 10 degrees flexion; the cast was continued for a subsequent six months' period to maintain the improved position. Following this latter period, all casts and splints were discontinued; he was examined frequently in the outpatient clinic. The last examination occurred at the age of 13, eight years after the first evaluation. Left knee

motion was 0 to 145 degrees and motion within normal limits was present at hips, ankles, and the right knee. His recreational activities included swimming and bicycling, as well as sports appropriate for his age and interests. He has participated in the home transfusion program since 1970 (Fig. 6-31).

The management of the joint evidencing chronic effusion, minimal pain or discomfort, and little restriction of motion deserves special comment. Some of these joints appear to respond to brief courses of steroid medication, to prophylactic concentrate infusion, to periods of mobilization or immobilization, to aspiration, or to empirically applied combinations of these measures. Other joints respond to none of these approaches; the synovitis perpetuates for prolonged periods of time with subsequent joint deterioration, motion restriction, and a reflex inhibition of muscle action (Figs. 6-32 and 6-33).[10] Better criteria appear

Figure 6-32. Capsular distention and condyle irregularity in seven year old.

Figure 6-33. Extensive destruction following three year perpetuating synovitis and eventual synovectomy.

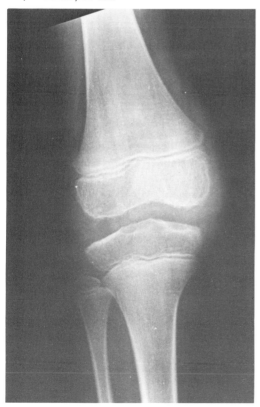

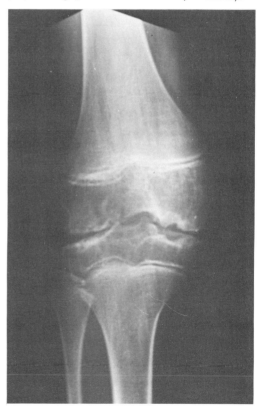

necessary to evaluate the on-going processes and to discriminate between the joints with apparent self-limiting problems and those which are nonresponsive to clinical management. The following case illustrates the former type of joint

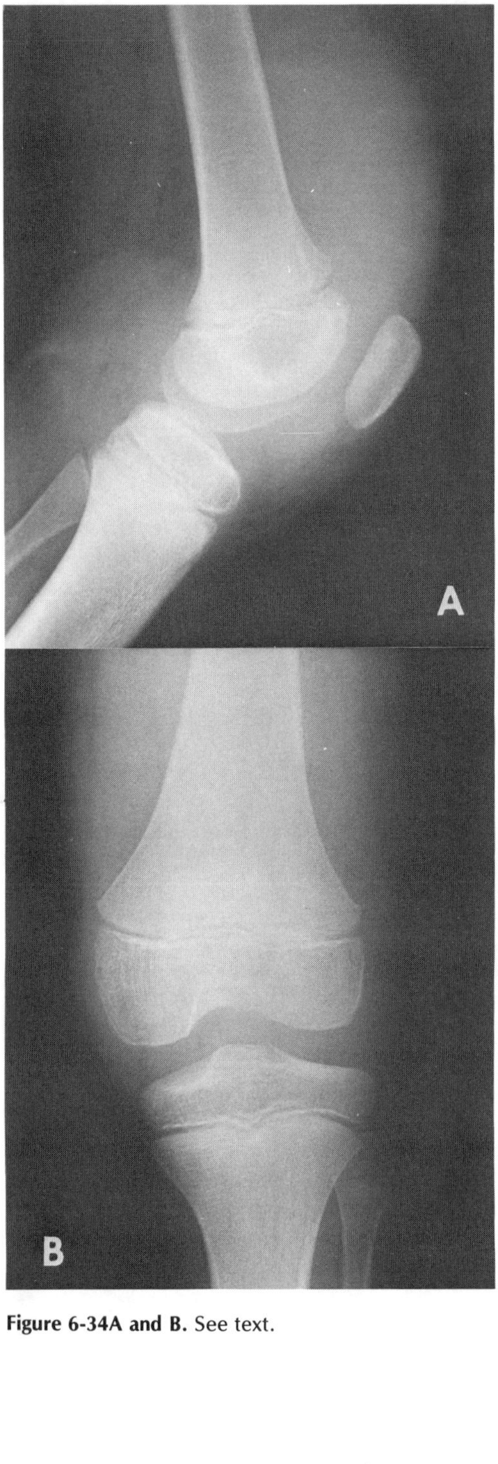

Figure 6-34A and B. See text.

which eventually responded to conservative management with minimal articular destruction:

A nine-year-old boy with less than 1 percent Factor VIII was seen initially in April 1971 for treatment of a hemarthrosis into the left knee. Reportedly, he had incurred a few episodes into the knee during the previous four or five years although normal joint motion and good thigh muscular development were apparent. The hemorrhage was treated with plasma concentrate daily for four days; a thermoplastic splint was used for supported walking. The knee was asymptomatic until January 1972 at which time marked effusion, pain, and restricted motion were present. Radiographically, the joint capsule appeared markedly distended; very minimal irregularity of the subchondral articular cortices of the femur were evident (Fig. 6-34 A and B). Arthrocentesis was performed under cover of plasma concentrate; the splint usage was resumed and exercise begun. One month later the knee evidenced a tense, nonpainful, extensive effusion which persisted for the next year with periodic increased or decreased severity. Six additional arthrocenteses, which produced from 20 to 145 ml of grossly bloody aspirate, were performed whenever increased fluid volume was apparent in the joint. Negative cultures were consistently obtained from the aspirated material. Eight courses of prednisolone of one week duration were administered during the year's period. In addition to therapeutic usage of plasma concentrate, daily prophylactic infusions were given for five periods varying from one week to one month in length; every other day transfusions were administered for one month. In summary, the patient was prophylaxed for one third of the year; inhibitor screening was negative. The thermoplastic splint was utilized for walking during most of the year; additionally, crutches were used when symptomatology increased. Swimming was

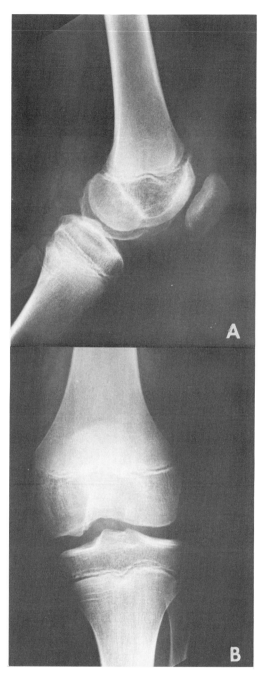

Figure 6-35A and B. See text.

creased to the fair range and knee motion was 15 to 120 degrees. Intramuscular injections of methylprednisolone acetate were given in January 1973 and prophylactic concentrate was administered daily for one month. By February, marked improvement was found of the synovial hypertrophy. Symptoms did not recur. In January 1974, synovitis was absent; the knees were equal in circumference. Motion of the left knee was 0 to 145 degrees; quadriceps strength was slightly less than normal. Radiographically, some thickening of the suprapatellar pouch was apparent; minimal irregularity of articular cortices of the femoral condyles was found (Fig. 6-35A and B).

Chronic Elbow Complaints

Ordinarily, elbow involvement begins in childhood with recurrent hemorrhage usually in the dominant arm. Initially, the proliferative synovium erodes the lateral margin of the olecranon; the olecranon deepens and the trochlea settles into the hollow with a resulting restriction of extension and flexion. Accelerated maturation, overgrowth, and premature closure of the epiphyseal centers occur. The radial head and the capitulum are prone to these changes producing limitation of forearm rotation. When elbow involvement begins in adolescence or early adulthood, after cessation of epiphyseal growth, diffuse loss of joint space and subchondral cyst formation occur, but the notching of the olecranon and the enlarged radial head are not found.[4] Muscle atrophy of arm and forearm musculature is readily apparent. The loss of rotary motion is more disabling than the loss of extension-flexion since many daily activities require supination and pronation.

The problems of chronic motion limitation, joint stiffness, and discomfort are not alleviated to any extent by the methods used to handle chronic knee complaints. Strengthening of elbow flexors and extensors as well as forearm musculature will provide some protection for the joint; however, attempts to con-

encouraged during the periods when acute problems were minimal. Exercise to the entire extremity, particularly emphasizing antigravity musculature, continued on the same basis. By December, quadriceps strength had de-

servatively decrease chronic motion restrictions are unsuccessful. Acquired am-
bidexterity is encouraged so the patient
can attempt to reduce the stress on the
symptomatic elbow. The periodic use of
the adjustable elbow splint may produce
some relief from episodic pain and discomfort.

Chronic Ankle and Foot Problems

Bleeding into the tibiotalar, fibulotalar,
and subtalar areas is frequent and, again,
initiates in childhood. Often the ankle
and the contralateral knee establish a cy-
clical pattern of hemorrhage. The loss of
dorsiflexion (ankle extension) is the earliest clinical finding and probably results
in part from fixation of the ankle in the
plantar-flexed position of comfort, during
recurrent hemorrhages. Altered joint
mechanics lead to slowly progressive
changes including the loss of joint space,
joint incongruity, and eventually the formation of marginal osteophytes, which
limit motion further. The foot may assume
a pronated position; hyperextension of
the metatarsophalangeal joints is common. Atrophy of the calf musculature is
usual and is coupled with decreased function of the tibialis anterior and the
peroneal group. The toe extensors, particularly the extensor digitorum longus,
appear to overfunction in an attempt to
produce dorsiflexion to compensate for
the dysfunction of the other ankle extensors. Hence, hammertoe deformities are
common.

A careful analysis of footwear is particularly important for patients with chronic
foot and ankle problems. Often selection
of proper shoes makes the difference between limited and unrestricted walking
ability. Shoes with rubber soles and flexible leather upper portions reaching above
the level of the malleoli are more easily
tolerated than those with leather soles and
rigid leather uppers. Lifts are added to
eliminate leg length inequality or to accommodate a rigid equinus position; arch
supports or sole and heel wedges are used
when clinically indicated. Custom molded
shoes are required when rigidly fixed de-

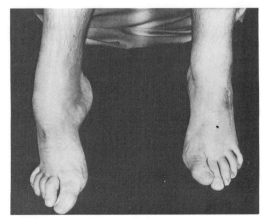

Figure 6-36. Rigidly fixed deformity of foot and
ankle.

formities as shown in Figure 6-36 preclude
commercial styles or when these produce
severe pressure areas.

The previously described laced canvas
and metal support is used to alleviate ankle
discomfort; however, a rigid leather lacer
may be required by those adult patients
who exhibit severe degenerative joint

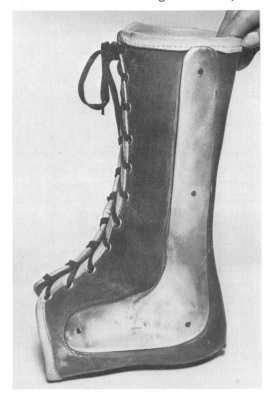

Figure 6-37. Rigid ankle support.

changes and symptomatically are unrelieved by footwear or the canvas support. This rigid model, fabricated on a mold of the foot, eliminates talar and subtalar motion (Fig. 6-37); its use is discontinued during periods when the ankles are asymptomatic.

Chronic Hip Manifestations

Hip involvement in hemophilia has several distinct patterns which appear to be related to the patient's age at the time of onset.[4] Problems in very early childhood are rare; however, intra-articular bleeding in the five to eight year old range produces radiographic changes indistinguishable from Legg-Perthes disease. Characteristically, these changes appear about six months after the hemorrhage. The course evolves like that of Perthes disease with the residual enlargement and "mushrooming" of the femoral head.[5] Consistent, close clinical and radiographic follow-up are important for several years after the initial insult. Rarely, bleeding into the young hip joint is severe enough to sublux or dislocate the femoral head. When this event occurs, it may be difficult to recognize and to treat and is extremely disabling.

This case history describes the typical course evolving from age four years, seven months when the patient, with less than 1 percent Factor IX, was admitted to the hospital for a three week period with an acute hemarthrosis of the right hip. Lyophilized plasma, traction, and exercise comprised the course of management. Initial radiographic changes were detected in the hip approximately eight months following the hemarthrosis. Over the next three years, a course of dissolution and subsequent reconstitution of the femoral head was observed (Fig. 6-38). During that period of time no complaints of pain, discomfort, or dysfunction were referable to the hip. Bleeding episodes into the hip were absent. Eight years after the original hemarthrosis, all motions of the right hip were within nor-

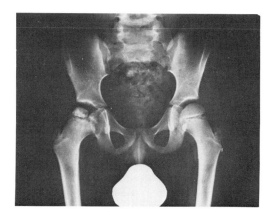

Figure 6-38. See text.

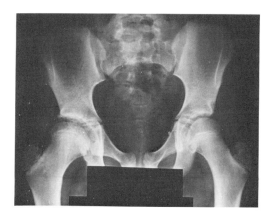

Figure 6-39. See text.

mal limits except for a slight reduction of internal rotation and radiographs show reformation of the femoral head (Fig. 6-39). During this period of time the patient was ambulatory without crutches, swam regularly, and routinely engaged in a daily exercise program to maintain strength of hip abductor and extensor groups.

Hip disease in the adult patient has subtle beginnings and only produces disability after many years' duration. A history of soft tissue swelling about the joint is frequent but that of a distinct hemarthrosis may be absent. Involvement begins in the superior weight bearing area with a portion of the head appearing to undergo avascular necrosis. Cystic changes appear in the head and adjacent acetabulum with loss of joint space. With aging, there may be either progressive resorption of the femoral head with proximal and lateral migration, or the joint space may be lost and extreme marginal osteophytoses may form.[4]

These hips are greatly restricted in motion and produce considerable pain and discomfort. Ambulation and other daily activity may be severely limited. When the hip involvement is coupled with knee and ankle dysfunction, the patient is severely disabled. Weight control is very important for these patients. Protection of the joint may be necessary through the use of canes or crutches while a wheelchair may be the most functional and energy conserving mechanism for some patients. Surgical reconstruction appears to offer the only solution to these problems of unremitting pain and increasing disability.

GENERAL CONCEPTS IN MANAGING MUSCULOSKELETAL PROBLEMS

Since hemophilia is a life-long disease, chronic and variable in nature, with acute problems superimposed on chronic ones, rehabilitation is viewed as a life-long process. Development of appropriate, consistent exercise habits is especially important at a young age for their carry over into adult life. Patients should stay in an optimum physical condition through specific exercise programs as well as recreational endeavors such as swimming, bicycling, golfing, tennis, and like activities. Most patients observe that fewer bleeding episodes occur when they are in better physical condition.

Starting at a young age, patients should be encouraged to learn their own physical abilities. Parents cannot do this for their child although many mothers and fathers make an attempt to impose unrealistic limitations on the young boy. Children should be allowed to experiment to discover what they can do and to learn from this experience. The experience deprived youth may develop into an emotionally deprived adult afraid to assume his place in society.

The assistive devices previously delineated are part of the total treatment program and not an end in themselves. They are used in combination with an appropriate exercise program and are utilized only for the minimum time required to obtain correction or to support the extremity. Relatively normal function of muscles and joints is impossible when the limb is enclosed in a double upright brace; therefore, bracing has been eliminated from this program which stresses activity and normal functioning.

Specific Exercise Considerations

The same kinds of exercise and exercise equipment are used with the hemophiliac as with other patients with similar musculoskeletal problems. The program includes the entire body, not just the most frequently involved joint. *Gradual* progression of the program is essential to minimize joint and muscle discomfort. Strengthening of antagonist muscles is preferred to passive stretching since the latter will produce involuntary contraction of those muscles placed under stretch. Weights, pulleys, and other devices for applying resistance are valuable when the patient is ready for resistive exercise. Treadmills are used to advantage to increase walking endurance and to practice proper gait patterns (Fig. 6-40); stationary bicycles provide effective joint mobilization when knee motion allows complete excursion of the pedals (Fig. 6-41). As mentioned previously, pro-

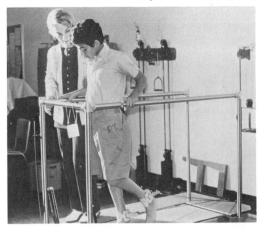

Figure 6-40. Treadmill walking with pulley resistance.

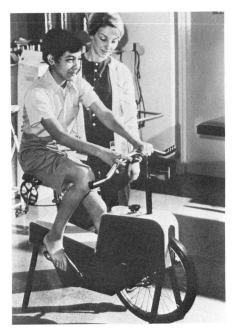

Figure 6-41. Using stationary bicycle.

phylactic use of plasma products prior to exercise prevents episodes of minor bleeding which will hinder advancement of the regimen. During an acute bleeding episode, exercise to the involved limb is discontinued; however, exercise to other body parts continues. Pain is the principal factor to determine when the subacutely involved limb can resume exercise.

When patients have had little experience with exercise or perhaps have experienced bleeding episodes from previous exercise attempts, sufficient time is spent in explaining the purpose and importance of various exercises. Definition and reiteration of treatment goals are significant at this initial encounter and a prompt follow-up appointment is essential to review any problems or questions which have arisen. Treatment goals usually include: (1) decrease deformity by increasing joint motion and muscle strength, (2) relieve pain or discomfort, (3) decrease the recovery period following a hemorrhage, (4) encourage maximum daily activity to maintain good muscle strength, and (5) determine the need for assistive devices. Patients are cautioned to expect some degree of muscle discom-

fort following the initiation of exercise so that discomfort is not immediately interpreted as pain of a hemorrhage. Vigorous programs, which are directed toward device-free ambulation in patients previously confined to wheelchairs or to long-term use of long leg braces, include both pool and dry land resistive exercise for two to three hours daily. When initial treatment goals have been attained, the exercise program becomes a maintenance one performed at home with periodic supervision from the physical therapist. Options are included which allow for disease variability; the number and type of exercises is kept to the reasonable amount which can be performed realistically by the patient in the course of his activity filled day.

Use of the Swimming Pool

A swimming pool is an ideal environment for exercise, alone or to supplement a dry land exercise program. Mobilization is accomplished with less strain on joints, with less pain, and with greater ease of movement. All hemophilic patients should be encouraged to learn to swim and to do so as often as possible (Fig. 6-42). During cold weather or periods when the pool is unheated, a wet suit such as used by skin divers can provide protection. Access to a pool is particularly important for those postsurgical patients whose convalescent period requires

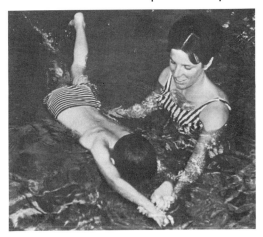

Figure 6-42. Seven year old learns to swim.

mobilization, those recovering from iliopsoas or retroperitoneal hemorrhage, and those with multiple chronic arthritic joint problems. A detailed manual of the theory and technique of exercise in the pool is available for guidance in establishing an underwater therapy program.[11]

Ideal water temperature is between 88 and 96°F. Warmer water tends to be debilitating when swimming or exercising for any length of time; colder water may cause aching and discomfort in the joints of some patients. Patients should be cautioned to avoid excessive exercise on the first day they enter the pool since ease of movement in the water may promote more activity than a joint or limb can tolerate initially.

Ambulation in the water may precede dry land walking, particularly in postsurgical and postiliopsoas hemorrhage patients. Walking begins in water of chest depth to reduce stress on the lower extremities and progresses to shallower depths in a few days' time; crutches can be weighted for water usage (Fig. 6-43). Gradual discontinuation of braces or supportive casts and splints is begun in the pool when the patient has been confined in these devices for an extended period (Fig. 6-44).

Hydroexercise is indicated following

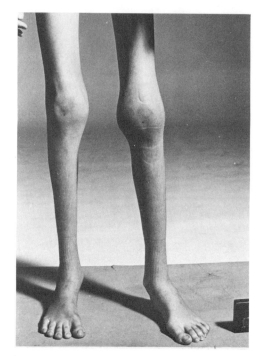

Figure 6-44. Legs of a twelve-year-old boy, who used bilateral Hessing braces for eight years. He began exercise program in pool and eventually was able to tolerate dry land exercise and device-free ambulation.

acute knee hemarthrosis when the need exists to mobilize the joint and to strengthen muscles of the involved limb as well as the rest of the body. As previously noted, participation in a pool program is important following iliopsoas hemorrhage. Management of multiple areas of chronic joint restriction and muscle weakness is enhanced when a pool is available. Particular benefit is noted by those adult patients with chronic complaints of joint stiffness, gelling, and discomfort coupled with a sedentary life style and decreased ability to perform activities such as walking.

Patients with Inhibitors

Diagnosis of an inhibitor should not mean mandatory exclusion from an exercise program. Indeed, the need for strong musculature is most important for these patients. The same techniques are used with them as with all other patients, however, progression from simple to more

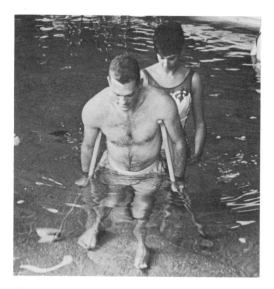

Figure 6-43. Crutch ambulation in water.

strenuous activity will proceed more slowly. Isometric exercises can be instituted as soon as an involved area shows decreased pain and swelling from the recent hemorrhage. Contract-relax techniques at several positions within the pain-free arc of motion are effective in obtaining maximal muscle contraction with minimal joint irritation.

Usually active exercise in the water precedes a dry land program. Hydroexercise, alone, is continued for a longer period of time for the inhibitor patient, for example for a two or three week period. If exercise is cautiously started and conscientiously followed, allowing for the interruptions of some hemorrhages, progression to a vigorous program is possible. Inhibitor patients are strongly urged to learn to swim since this activity provides a recreational opportunity while reducing the possibility of trauma from body contact. These patients are encouraged to be as normally active as possible. The majority of our children with inhibitors engage in ordinary playground and peer-play activities.

When supportive devices are necessary, they may be used for longer periods of time. For example, the thermoplastic leg splint may be worn for one or two months following recurrences of knee hemorrhage. Since the condition of the inhibitor patient may change frequently because of bleeding which cannot be controlled by routine measures, the treatment program must be adapted accordingly. Any therapist treating these patients must be sensitive to this variability and determine each treatment period if changes have occurred which necessitate altering the program. The therapist should avoid discouragement when the inhibitor patient must temporarily suspend part of his exercise program because of bleeding episodes. Such discouragement is conveyed, overtly or subtly, to the patient who is already troubled by the refractory nature of his condition.

Postsurgical Mobilization

Generally, postsurgical management, including use of exercise and initiation of weight bearing, is comparable to that of the nonhemophilic person having the same surgical procedure although with some procedures, such as total hip arthroplasty, protection from stress may be extended slightly. As indicated in prior chapters, plasma concentrates are infused on a daily basis for a 14 day period to attain minimal factor levels of 30 percent. When exercise programs continue beyond the two week period, concentrate is administered prior to exercise. Periods of complete immobilization are reduced to a minimum time period because of the frequency of multiple joint involvement and the resultant stiffness from inactivity. When needed, exercise to the unoperated extremities begins on the second or third postoperative day as the patient's medical status allows. Presurgical orientation to the postsurgical exercise program proves beneficial in early mobilization of the patient. Pool therapy is frequently used to mobilize the limb following removal of casts, to initiate walking following surgery, and to provide some general body conditioning after surgical confinement.

RECREATIONAL ACTIVITIES

Questions arise frequently from parents as well as school and health personnel about the kinds of activities or sports in which a hemophilic boy can engage. Some boys have been encouraged to participate in all or part of a school's physical education program; others have been arbitrarily banned from playgrounds by school personnel based on their medical diagnosis. The uniqueness of each boy must be considered in planning a physical activity program for him since each individual differs in his physical abilities, the severity of his musculoskeletal problems, the incidence of his bleeding episodes, and most importantly in his likes and dislikes. Counsel with the boy and his parents should be sought in establishing a physical activity program since he will be able to delineate fully the activities in which he engages now, and those which he wants to undertake.

In general, certain sports are encouraged; tennis, golf, badminton, cycling, and swimming are pursued successfully by a large number of hemophilic children and adults. A number of our patients have played Little League baseball; some participate in intramural basketball, soccer, and other sports. Vigorous contact sports including football or basketball, are not encouraged, however, the final decision to participate in these sports rests with the patient and his parents. They should be appraised of the specific risks and what these mean in terms of potentially life-threatening or crippling problems so that a decision is based on informed reality and not emotional conjecture. Younger children should be allowed to participate in playground activities to afford them the opportunity to join with classmates in usual play experiences. Again, common sense and consultation with the boy and his parents will provide practical guides for activities.

Contact between the physical therapist at the Center and the physical education teacher is helpful for the incorporation of specific exercises into the hemophiliac's physical education program when this is possible. The school can assume an important role by encouraging boys with hemophilia to establish patterns of physical activity to keep themselves in good physical condition, now and for their future.

SUMMARY

The residuals of hemorrhage into joint and soft tissue areas of the extremities present the major problems of disability found in these coagulation disorders.

Three pathologic processes appear to combine to produce classic arthropathy: hemorrhage and the responding synovitis, the degeneration of the articular cartilage, and the formation of subchondral cysts. Nonsurgical management of the musculoskeletal problems is based upon the adequate treatment of each bleeding episode, the utilization of exercise to normalize function, the use of temporary dynamic splints, and the care-

ful, on-going evaluation of the musculoskeletal status of each patient.

Hopefully, this treatment approach will greatly reduce the crippling sequelae for those patients managed in this manner since their childhood and perhaps decrease some of the disabling manifestations found in the adult.

In addition to the infusion of plasma concentrates, acute hemarthroses may be managed with immobilization and/or arthrocentesis. Considerable attention is directed toward the management of the sequelae of knee hemarthroses because of the frequent occurrence of this bleeding as well as the treatment of elbow and ankle episodes. Certain soft tissue hemorrhages are precursors to the development of long standing deformity; areas of concern include the forearms, the calf musculature, and the iliopsoas muscle group. Exercise and daily activity, such as walking, should be initiated cautiously following the acute episode with attention directed toward the sensory and the motor status of the involved extremity.

The chronic joint degeneration found with repeated hemarthroses presents challenges to management, particularly as the patient grows older. Exercise and corrective or supportive devices are utilized in conservative management, however, surgical intervention may be the only course available for restoration of function in the patient with severe joint involvement.

Rehabilitation of the hemophilic patient should be considered a life-long process since acute problems become superimposed on chronic manifestations. Patients should be counseled to maintain their bodies in good condition through specific exercise as well as recreational endeavors. The same kinds of exercise and exercise equipment are used with the hemophiliac as with other patients with comparable musculoskeletal problems. Hydroexercise and swimming are particularly beneficial. When initiating an exercise regimen or increasing the intensity of an existing one, plasma concentrate is infused prior to exercise to prevent any bleeding which could be precipitated by vigorous activity.

Recreational or sports endeavors should be planned with the hemophilic boy and his parents keeping in mind the boy's physical abilities, the incidence of his bleeding episodes, the severity of existing musculoskeletal problems, and his wishes.

The availability of a physical therapist or other musculoskeletal expert is important when the staffing of a hemophilia center is planned. Thus, joint and muscle function can be evaluated following acute bleeding episodes and the musculoskeletal status of each patient can be followed on a longitudinal basis. Dysfunctions can be identified and appropriate corrective measures can be instituted promptly.

Since the pathologic pathways producing hemophilic arthropathy are poorly understood, research efforts are needed to better delineate the histochemical and biochemical processes; such study could provide a more scientific framework for the clinical management. Additionally, better definition of the kinesiologic impacts of some of the common deformities could place the treatment of these deformities on a more objective basis.

REFERENCES

1. Weiss, A. E., and Brinkhous, K. M.: Hemarthroses and hemarthropathy in hemophilia A and B, in McCollough, N. C. III (ed.): *Comprehensive Management of Musculoskeletal Disorders in Hemophilia*. National Academy of Sciences, Washington, D.C., 1973.
2. Hilgartner, M. W.: Pathogenesis of joint changes in hemophilia, in McCollough, N. C. III. (ed.): *Comprehensive Management of Musculoskeletal Disorders in Hemophilia*. National Academy of Sciences, Washington, D.C., 1973.
3. De Palma, A. F., and Cotter, J.: Hemophilic arthropathy. Clin. Orthop. 8:163–189, 1956.
4. Martinson, A.: Personal communication, 1974.
5. Caffey, J.: *Pediatric X-Ray Diagnosis*, ed. 5. Year Book Medical Publisher, Chicago, 1967.
6. Knott, M., and Voss, D.: *Proprioceptive Neuromuscular Facilitation*. Harper and Row, New York, 1956.
7. Boone, D. C., Greenberg, R., Perry, J., and Dietrich, S. L.: The energy expenditure of walking in hemophilic patients with knee motion restriction. Presentation at annual conference, American Physical Therapy Association, 1975.
8. Goodfellow, J., Fearn, C. B. d'A., and Matthews, J. M.: Iliacus haematoma. A common complication of hemophilia. J. Bone Joint Surg. 49B:748–756, 1967.
9. *Joint Motion: Method of Measuring and Recording*. American Academy of Orthopaedic Surgeons, Chicago, 1963.
10. Boone, D. C.: Studies of joint motion in hemophilia, in McCollough, N.C. III. (ed.): *Comprehensive Management of Musculoskeletal Disorders in Hemophilia*. National Academy of Sciences, Washington, D.C., 1973.
11. De Andrade, J. R., Grant, C., and Dixon, A. St. J.: Joint distention and reflex muscle inhibition in the knee. J. Bone Joint Surg. 47A:313, 1965.
12. Lowman, C. L., and Roen, S. G.: *Underwater Therapy*. Orthopaedic Foundation Publisher, Los Angeles, 1961.

SUGGESTED READINGS

Ahlberg, A.: Haemophilia in Sweden VII. Incidence, treatment and prophylaxis of arthropathy and other musculoskeletal manifestations of haemophilia A and B. Acta Orthop. Scand. No. 77, 1965.

Duthie, R. B., Matthews, J. M., Rizza, C. R., and Steel, W. M.: *The Management of Musculoskeletal Problems in the Haemophilias*. Blackwell Scientific Publications, Oxford, 1972.

Kerr, C. B.: *The Management of Hemophilia*. Australian Medical Publishing Co., Glebe, Australia, 1963.

7

SURGICAL MANAGEMENT OF MUSCULOSKELETAL PROBLEMS

Jordan M. Rhodes and Alice M. Martinson

GENERAL CONSIDERATIONS

A hemophilic patient should not be considered a surgical candidate unless adequate supplies of plasma concentrate are available for intraoperative and postoperative coverage and unless facilities for postoperative musculoskeletal rehabilitation are easily accessible to the patient. Participation in a self-infusion program is advantageous for the postsurgical convalescence. Best results will be obtained by a team conversant with hemophilia and including the hematologist, the orthopedist, nursing staff, physical and occupational therapists, psychologists, family and vocational/educational counselors.

MEDICAL CONSIDERATIONS

Major surgery may be performed on hemophiliacs with safety if clotting factor concentrates are administered in sufficient quantities to achieve plasma factor levels of approximately 100 percent at the initiation of a procedure. Levels are maintained at a daily minimum of 30 percent for the first two postoperative weeks. These levels are possible only if the patient does not have a circulating inhibitor; thus, the presence of an inhibitor is an *absolute contraindication* to elective surgery, and the patient's response to replacement therapy must be ascertained prior to surgery. We consider Factor IX deficiency to be a relative contraindication to elective surgery since we have experienced a large number of thromboembolic phenomena in patients requiring large quantities of Factor IX concentrate. This thromboembolic potential is believed due to the presence of other activated clotting factors in the material as previously discussed in Chapter 2 where further details about hematologic management of surgical patients can be found.

The patient should be carefully evaluated prior to surgery for the presence of concurrent disease, especially convulsive disorders and hepatitis, as well as tendencies toward drug dependence or addiction. The surgeon and the anesthesiologist should be aware of all current medications which the patient is consuming. Accessibility of adequate venous pathways should be ascertained presurgically.

Because of the large quantities of concentrates and blood transfusions which may be required, the risk of serum induced hepatitis is very high. The history of prior episodes of hepatitis should be carefully sought since the halogenated ether anesthetics must not be used on those cases.

Postoperatively, larger than usual dosages of analgesics and sedatives may be required since many surgical candidates have been using analgesics regularly preoperatively and have developed a tolerance to them. Rarely, true drug dependency occurs; however, this should be known preoperatively so that withdrawal reactions can be avoided. Salicylate containing analgesics alter the coagulability of the blood as well as the patient's response to infused concentrates and should be avoided. Additionally, the patient should withdraw preoperatively from any other medications which may interfere with the coagulation mechanism, i.e., indomethacin.

Following this protocol, 163 major surgical procedures have been performed since 1968; 113 of these were orthopedic procedures. We have had no loss of limb, an overall infection rate of 3.7 percent, and one death secondary to pulmonary embolus following emergency abdominal surgery in a patient with Factor IX deficiency.

SURGICAL CONSIDERATIONS

Surgical treatment of musculoskeletal problems in hemophiliacs may be undertaken to relieve pain and recurrent bleeding as well as to improve function when nonsurgical methods have been unsuccessful. The patient and physician must be fully aware of the multitude of risks involved, and resources must be available for handling any problem which may arise.

The effects of general inactivity should be anticipated since these tend to be greater in the hemophilic patient with his usual multiple arthritic problems. Nonoperated limbs should be mobilized rapidly and general body immobility kept to a minimum during the postoperative period. Rehabilitative efforts should be continued under prophylactic factor administration until musculoskeletal function is sufficient to protect the limb from exercise trauma with subsequent bleeding.

The following types of surgical procedures have been performed on patients at this Center: arthroplasties, both excisional and replacement; synovectomies; osteotomies; arthrodeses; contracture releases; decompressions of compartment syndromes and peripheral nerves; excision of pseudotumors; and fracture management using both closed and open reduction.

Specific Procedures

EXCISIONAL ARTHROPLASTY OF THE ELBOW. This procedure is indicated after epiphys-

eal maturation to improve elbow and forearm function and to relieve pain associated with degenerative arthritic changes and recurrent bleeding. A radial head resection and partial synovectomy are performed. Minimal postoperative immobilization is used; range of motion exercises are begun within 72 hours postoperatively. This procedure has been very successful in providing pain relief and in reducing the incidence of hemarthrosis. Motion, principally forearm rotation, has improved also with the improvement being maintained for a follow-up period of several years. The following case history describes multiple surgical procedures in one patient; the first of these was a radial head excision.

From early childhood, this man with severe Factor VIII deficiency had experienced recurrent intra-articular bleeding into both elbows and the right knee. At age 28, the right elbow became increasingly stiff and painful with frequent bleeding episodes. No improvement was noted with conservative management, i.e., regular concentrate infusion, splinting, and indomethacin. Joint

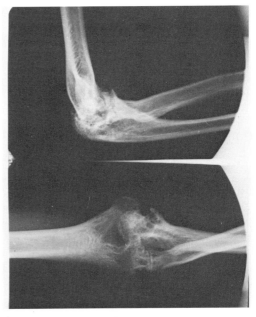

Figure 7-1. Presurgical roentgenogram of radial head excision.

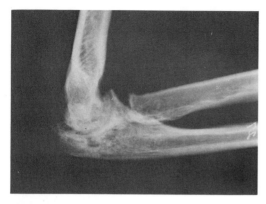

Figure 7-2. Postsurgical roentgenogram of radial head excision.

motion at that time was extension-flexion from 35 to 120 degrees, forearm pronation of 5 degrees, and supination of 0 degrees. In March 1970, a right radial head excision and subtotal synovectomy were performed. His postsurgical course was uneventful with eight days' hospitalization; 12,750 units of Factor VIII concentrate were administered. In the four years since surgery, he has had no bleeding episodes into the elbow nor has he had pain in that joint. Range of motion is extension-flexion from 25 to 130 degrees, 10 degrees of pronation, and no supination (Figs. 7-1 and 7-2).

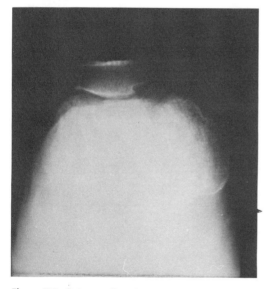

Figure 7-3. Preoperative view.

In early 1973, he noted increasing crepitus, swelling, and retropatellar pain in the right knee. During the next year, these symptoms failed to respond to indomethacin, exercise, and regular concentrate administration. In March 1974, a patellectomy of the right knee was performed. Preoperative joint motion was from 15 to 105 degrees. He was unable to extend his knee against resistance because of severe retropatellar pain; the right thigh was 5 cm smaller than the left in circumference. His walking ability was restricted markedly (Fig. 7-3).

At surgery, extensive degeneration of the articular surfaces of the patella and the distal femur were noted. He was hospitalized for 11 days and used 31,414 units of Factor VIII concentrate. After three weeks of cast immobilization, he began intensive exercises to strengthen antigravity musculature. Six months postoperatively he has only occasional right knee pain; he is ambulatory for unlimited distances without support. He has regained his preoperative range of knee motion and has only 1.5 cm residual right thigh atrophy.

HIP ARTHROPLASTY. This is a major undertaking in the hemophiliac because of the extensive arthritic changes and soft tissue fibrosis secondary to chronic hemorrhage. Cup arthroplasty has been uniformly disappointing and total hip replacement is now considered the procedure of choice for disabling hip involvement. The Charnley-Muller prosthesis has been used in all cases in our series. The operative technique and postoperative management are essentially the same as in nonhemophiliacs. Operating time and intraoperative blood loss are much greater than normal because of the extensive periarticular fibrosis, so that concentrate replacement during the procedure is necessary. (Refer to Chap. 2 for further details.) Careful observation is essential for any postoperative hemorrhage which may sublux or dislocate the femoral component.

In general, rehabilitation should be accomplished at a slower pace and weight bearing protected by crutches or a cane for a longer period in order to minimize the occurrence and extent of deep tissue bleeding. If a pool is available, the water is an ideal environment for initiating ambulation on the fifth or sixth postoperative day.

The following case histories detail total hip replacements for fracture management and coincidental with iliac pseudotumor excision.

A 22-year-old man with severe Factor VIII deficiency suddenly developed severe left hip pain and physically collapsed while hiking. A history was elicited of mild hip discomfort during the preceding five or six months. Admission radiographs revealed a displaced subcapital fracture of the left femoral neck (Fig. 7-4) and degenerative changes in the joint (Fig. 7-5). Because of the pre-existing arthritic disease in the hip and the great likelihood of subsequent avascular necrosis of the head fragment, primary total hip replacement was the treatment of choice.

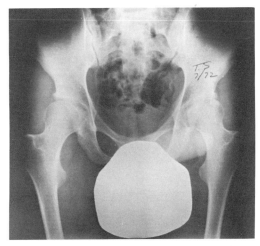

Figure 7-5. Pre-existing arthritic disease, four months prior to fracture.

At surgery the hip capsule was very thick and fibrotic; the femoral head was devoid of articular cartilage and had multiple small subchondral cysts. A Charnley-Muller prosthesis was inserted. The total operating time was 4.5 hours with a blood loss of 3000 ml. His postoperative course was complicated by temperature elevation for the first six days, but his wound healed primarily. During the one month of hospitalization, 76,500 units of Factor VIII concentrate were used.

At his 18 month postoperative evaluation, he reported minimal discomfort in

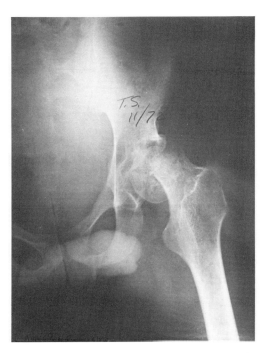

Figure 7-4. Displaced subcapital fracture of the femoral neck.

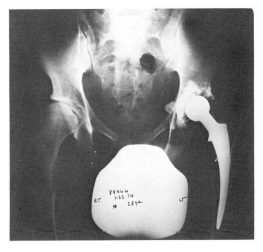

Figure 7-6. Twenty-six months postsurgically.

the hip and had resumed 10 mile hikes. He was able to ascend and descend stairs without difficulty and to put on and take off his shoes and socks in a normal manner. He believed that his functional range of motion was essentially the same as before the fracture. He has incurred no bleeding episodes into the hip. A postsurgical roentgenogram at 26 months is shown in Figure 7-6.

When this 56-year-old patient with severe Factor VIII deficiency was first seen at this Center in 1972, he had a large left flank and buttock mass. Radiographs revealed a large destructive lesion of the iliac wing and severe degenerative changes in the left hip (Fig. 7-7). History indicated that at age

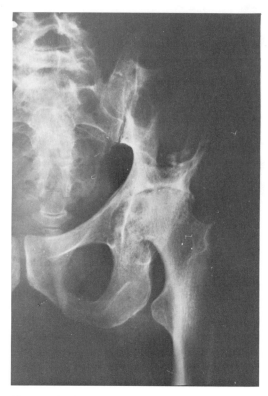

Figure 7-8. Roentgenogram immediately prior to surgery.

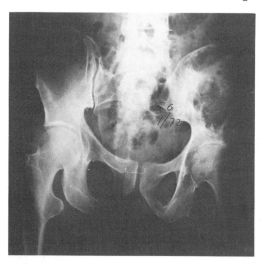

Figure 7-7. Roentgenogram 18 months before surgery.

16 he had undergone open surgical drainage of what proved to be a left retroperitoneal hematoma. Despite massive blood loss he survived that procedure. The radiographic report from that hospitalization mentioned a lytic lesion in the left acetabular roof. During the next 40 years, he experienced gradually increasing pain and stiffness in the left hip.

In June 1973, because of intolerable hip pain and documented enlargement

of the mass, he underwent excision of a large iliac pseudotumor and a Charnley-Muller total hip replacement (Fig. 7-8). At surgery, the pseudotumor was found to occupy the entire iliac fossa and was continuous through an

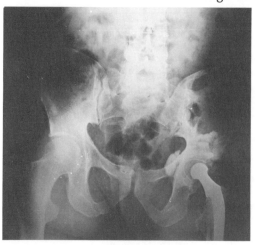

Figure 7-9. One year postsurgical evaluation.

iliac defect with the mass in the buttock. His postoperative course was difficult and required 15 units of whole blood, 125,200 units of Factor VIII concentrate, and seven weeks' hospitalization. Postoperatively, he had dramatic relief of hip pain. When seen for his one year postsurgical evaluation, significant increases in hip motion were apparent (Fig. 7-9). No bleeding episodes had occurred into the hip, buttock, or pelvic areas. He walked without support for unlimited distances and had returned to his previous business endeavors. The iliac defect, which was not bone grafted, had not changed; there was no evidence of recurrence of the pseudotumor.

DEBRIDEMENT ARTHROPLASTY. This procedure is indicated when a joint with good functional potential is being compromised by osteophytic formation. The anterior talotibial articular margin is frequently involved with a resultant painful mechanical block to good ankle motion. Meniscus disease may be mimicked by para-articular femoral condyle osteophytes. Partial synovectomy is performed simultaneously with the debridement; weight bearing is initiated in 48 to 72 hours. Institution and progression of exercise depends upon the specific joint and extent of the surgical procedure.

SYNOVECTOMY. Synovectomy is indicated in the presence of chronic synovitis unresponsive to medical management with minimal apparent destruction of articular surfaces and good joint motion. Postoperatively a compression wrap is applied and weight bearing is begun on the second or third postoperative day. Gentle gravity manipulation is performed under general anesthesia on the seventh postoperative day; active joint motion is begun after the manipulation. Because of the variability and unpredictability of the natural history of hemophilic arthropathy, more specific indications for synovectomy are at this point unclear. However, younger individuals are now being considered for this procedure in an attempt to arrest the degenerative process at an early stage. In older individuals with more extensive joint changes but a relatively good range of motion, synovectomy may be accompanied by debridement of the menisci and excision of marginal osteophytes as previously discussed.

PATELLECTOMY. When painful knee motion is accompanied by findings suggestive of patellofemoral arthritis, patellectomy is useful. This procedure should not be performed at the same time as synovectomy or joint debridement since the early mobilization essential for success in the latter procedures cannot be accomplished, and severe arthrofibrosis and marked motion loss will result. Ambulation in a long leg cast is begun within the first postoperative week and the cast maintained for three to four weeks before mobilization is begun.

OSTEOTOMY. Osteotomy is used to correct or improve functional musculoskeletal alignment and is most commonly performed about the knee for the treatment of fixed flexion deformities. Concomitant angular and rotational deformities may be corrected at the same time. Fixation is accomplished with heavy threaded Steinmann pins. The extension desubluxation hinged cast described in Chapter 6 should be used preoperatively to lengthen the posterior neurovascular structures.

ARTHRODESIS. This procedure has been used sparingly and only in those circumstances where a stiff joint is intolerably painful. Its best application would seem to be at the tibial talar joint where fusion can provide a stable, painless, plantigrade foot. Healing of the arthrodeses has been prompt and uncomplicated as described in the following case history.

At age 25 years, this patient with severe Factor VIII deficiency noted increasing pain, stiffness, and hemarthroses in the left ankle. Two years later his ankle pain was so severely disabling that he was unable to walk more than a few feet. He had developed a severe drug dependency problem. At that time, the ankle evidenced a 10 degree

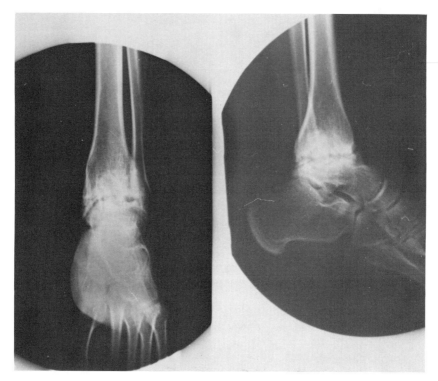

Figure 7-10. Presurgical roentgenograms.

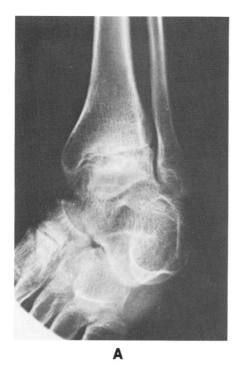

A

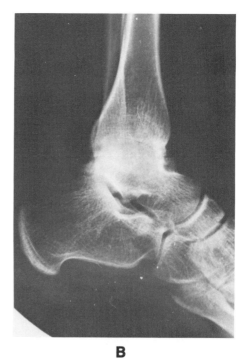

B

Figure 7-11A and B. Eight months postsurgically.

equinus contracture and had only a few degrees of painful motion (Fig. 7-10). In February 1970, a tibial talar arthrodesis was performed with supplemental iliac bone grafting. The postoperative course was complicated by infection at the iliac donor site which responded to drainage and antibiotic administration. He was hospitalized for 29 days and used 37,250 units of Factor VIII plasma concentrate during his postsurgical convalescence. His arthrodesis united in 12 weeks (Figs. 7-11A and B). Three years later, he is able to hike approximately five miles in rough terrain without pain; he is employed full time in a rural area as manager of a camping facility. He has resolved his problems of drug dependency.

ISOLATED SOFT TISSUE RELEASES. These are indicated infrequently and only in younger patients. Usually contractures are associated with such significant remodeling of joint surfaces that the desired amount of change in joint position cannot be obtained with soft tissue surgery alone. Posterior knee or ankle release may be required, however, in conjunction with realignment osteotomies.

DECOMPRESSION OF PERIPHERAL NERVES. This procedure has rarely been required. Recurrent hemorrhage into a chronically arthritic elbow may produce sufficient ulnar nerve compression so that anterior transposition is necessary to preserve function. Hemorrhage into the carpal canal may imperil the median nerve. Although we have not found it necessary in this clinic, a carpal tunnel release would seem indicated if progressive loss of function is occurring despite appropriate concentrate administration and immobilization. A similar comment may be made about hemorrhage into the anterior tibial compartment. Femoral neuropathy is not unusual with severe iliopsoas hemorrhage; however, it has been our experience that resolution usually occurs with

time and attempted surgical treatment is not recommended.

ARTHROCENTESIS. Arthrocentesis is performed on any joint presenting severe acute distention, with or without pain, which compromises function. Plasma concentrate is administered to attain 50 percent levels upon completion of the aspiration. Steroid injections, used frequently in the past, are not recommended except in the unusual instance when chronic synovitis is a major component of the problem. The joint is immobilized for 24 hours following aspiration; concentrate is administered on the fifth postaspiration day to raise the circulating level to 20 percent. A more detailed description of the aspiration technique and subsequent rehabilitation procedures can be found in Chapters 4 and 6.

Management of Other Problems

Fractures should be managed in the same way as in nonhemophiliacs; however, adequate plasma concentrate should be administered as soon as the trauma is reported. When indicated, firm internal fixation will allow beneficial early mobilization of adjacent joints. Extreme care should be taken when circular plasters are applied over fresh fractures, however mild, and plasma concentrate should be administered for an appropriate time postfracture to manage the accompanying soft tissue injury. Infusion of plasma concentrate to achieve 50 percent levels is particularly important prior to cast changes while union is incomplete. Union of fractures proceeds at the same rate as in nonhemophilic patients; however, secure immobilization is essential to prevent recurrent hemorrhage at the fracture site. Often, soft tissue swelling following an acute fracture is extreme; great care should be taken to ensure that a snugly fitting cast is maintained as the swelling resolves. It should be kept in mind that a fracture may be a precursor to or result of a pseudotumor.

8

HEMOPHILIC PSEUDOTUMORS

Alice Martinson

Pseudotumors are an unusual and puzzling complication of severe coagulation disorders. The etiology of these pseudotumors remains somewhat unclear but Duthie believes that hemorrhage involving bone may occur in three situations: (1) subperiosteal hemorrhage; (2) intraosseous bleeding; and (3) bleeding into muscle with wide periosteal attachments.[1] Before the availability of concentrates these lesions carried a dismal prognosis, with persistent hemorrhage or sepsis and death routinely following attempts to aspirate or surgically drain them. In 1966, Gunning indicated a 75 to 80 percent mortality rate from surgical treatment.[2]

Since 1962, at this Center, 19 pseudotumors have been diagnosed in 14 patients with severe coagulation disorders; 13 had Factor VIII deficiency and one had Factor IX deficiency. One patient formed pseudotumors in nine bones. All these patients were less than 30 years old at the time of pseudotumor diagnosis except for a 56-year-old man with a large iliac lesion and hip symptomatology reported since adolescence. (See Chap. 7, p. 90.) No mortalities occurred among those patients treated here.

Diagnosis of these lesions depended upon clinical suspicion as well as radiographic confirmation. The usual presenting complaints were pain and localized swelling and tenderness. The majority of the surgically treated lesions were first diagnosed on routine screening joint radiographs. The sites of involvement were proximal tibia, 4; hindfoot, 4; mandible, 3; metacarpal/metatarsal, 3; and one each in the thigh, the ilium, the patella, the ulna, the distal humerus, and the proximal humerus.

The lesions in the extremities appeared to fall into one of two clinical types: those occurring in immature and those in mature bone. Nine occurred in the carpometacarpal or tarsometatarsal bones of skeletally immature individuals and pursued a florid course of pain and swelling with radiographic evidence of cortical expansion and extensive osteolysis. All these lesions resolved with immobilization, observation, and plasma infusion; however, cortical collapse and distortion were quite prominent in weight-bearing bones. Growth arrest was frequent.

The seven tumors in the major long bones developed in skeletally mature individuals, enlarged more slowly, and reached greater size before they were diagnosed. X-rays revealed an expansile lesion which was surrounded by a thin cortical shell giving the lesion a "soap bubble" appearance. Intralesional calcification was not prominent; progressive enlargement was the rule. Three of these tumors were related to the subchondral area of joints and radiographically resembled the degenerative cysts which are common in hemophilic arthropathy. Progressive enlargement resulted in surgical confirmation of their true nature. A recent review of pseudotumors from another large center has shown a distribution of lesions quite similar to ours.[3]

The histopathology of hemophilic pseudotumors has been well defined by Fernandez de Valderrama and Matthews.[4]

They noted three distinct zones within the lesions: a central gelatinous clot; an intermediate zone of loosely organized, fibrous tissue containing numerous small blood vessels and hemosideris pigment; and a tough fibrous outer zone containing both reticular and elastic fibers. When the cyst has involved muscle, the outer wall can also contain scattered atrophic muscle fibers. All lesions in this series which were biopsied demonstrate the triple layer configuration. Foreign body giant cells were seen infrequently. A striking feature of most lesions was the intense vascularity of the middle and outer zones.

The three mandibular lesions were associated with disordered tooth eruption or periodontal infections; their management is described in Chapter 10.

Rest, observation, and lyophilized plasma administration were the methods of treatment before the advent of the plasma concentrates. Low dosage irradiation was used twice on different lesions in one patient. All those tumors which were treated with plasma products, immobilization, and observation regressed spontaneously and healed. Daily concentrate administration appeared to accelerate the resolution process in those cases for which it was available. The two irradiated lesions resolved and remain healed for eight and five years, respectively. No essential difference in their course or result was evident when compared with other lesions in the same patient which were not irradiated. One large tibial lesion was irradiated elsewhere with 1600 roentgens. Arrest of the anterior portion of the proximal tibial epiphyseal plate occurred. While the lesion was temporarily arrested, enlargement resumed approximately three years later; surgical management was eventually required five years after irradiation. A large thigh lesion, associated with the nonunion of a femoral fracture, was diagnosed in a patient who returned to his home in a foreign country before treatment could be instituted. Subsequently, we learned of his fatal termination three years later from the progressive enlargement and catastrophic rupture of the lesion.

The following case history describes conservative management of multiple lesions:

This patient, with severe Factor VIII deficiency, first exhibited pseudotumor formation in 1962 at the age of eight years. The initial lesions were located in the right middle metacarpal (Fig. 8-1A) and the right first metatarsal. During the next three years, tumors formed in the right calcaneus and talus as well (Fig. 8-2). Progression, gradual regression, and reformation of all tumors occurred except the metacarpal lesion which demonstrated a continued healing process (Fig. 8-1B). In 1965, the left talus evidenced a tumor formation and subsequent destruction followed in 1966 by involvement of the left calcaneus and right humeral epicondyle and in 1967 by reactivation of the process in the right talus (Fig. 8-3). Bony defects from these later lesions were gradually filled; however, the humeral pseudotumor expanded again in 1968 with olecranon involvement (Figs. 8-4 and 8-5). The proximal phalanx of the right great toe became involved in 1968, also. By mid-1969, all pseudotumors showed healing and filling of the defects; by mid-1970, all were judged to be completely healed with bony deformation in most cases (Fig. 8-6). Since then, neither recurrences of tumors at the noted sites nor new lesion formations have been found. However, multiple bleeding episodes have occurred into soft tissue areas of the lower extremities as well as into ankles, knees, elbows, and the left shoulder.

Until 1968, management of the lesions was restricted to rest, plasma administration, and observation usually in the hospital. In fact, 296 days of in-hospital care were recorded for management of these multiple lesions during the six year period when pseudotumor formation was prevalent. Two of the pseudotumors, left talus (1965) and right elbow (1968), were irradiated with two treatments of 100 roentgens each. From 1965 until early 1968 this patient was confined to a wheel-

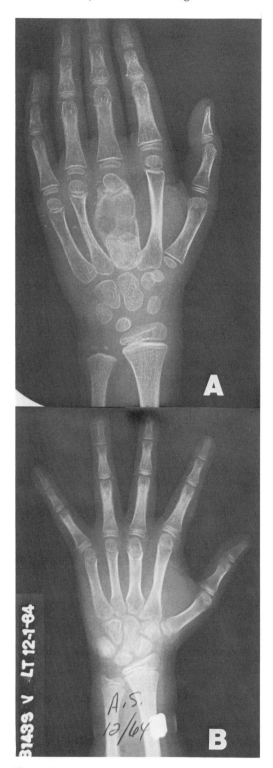

Figure 8-1. A, Pseudotumor, right middle metacarpal, 1962. B, Right hand two years later.

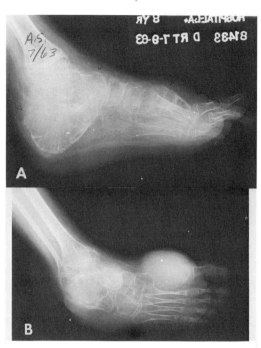

Figure 8-2. A, Right foot and ankle, July 1963. B, Expanded lesion of first metatarsal, December 1964.

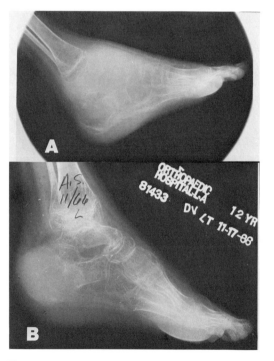

Figure 8-3. Left foot and ankle. A, May 1965; B, November 1966.

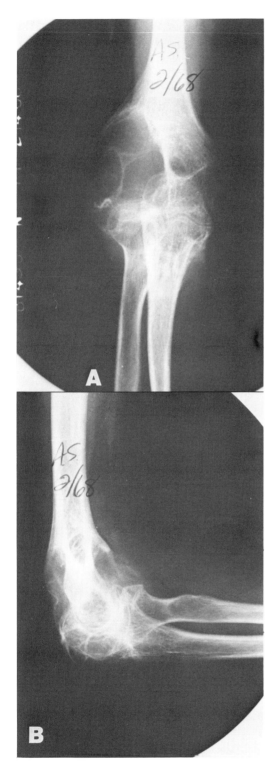

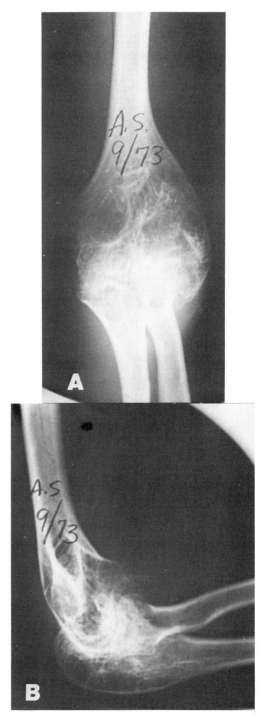

Figure 8-4A and B. Distal humeral-olecranon involvement, February 1968.

Figure 8-5A and B. Same areas as Figure 8-4, September 1973.

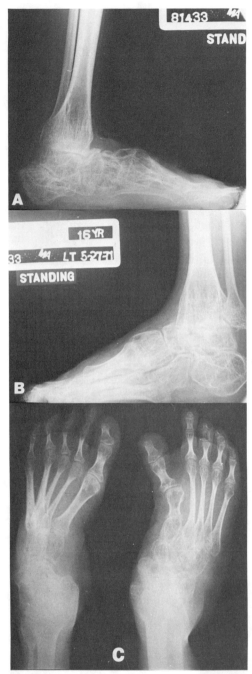

Figures 8-6. Standing views of (A) right, (B) left, and (C) both feet, May 1971.

chair; however, he received exercise almost continuously as an inpatient and outpatient to maintain joint mobility and muscle strength of body parts not involved in pseudotumor activity. In early 1968, he was hospitalized for intensive efforts directed toward ambulation; Factor VIII concentrate was administered on a prophylactic basis. Since then, he has been ambulatory without use of canes or crutches; currently, he utilizes custom-made bilateral polypropylene foot and ankle supports to stabilize his hind and forefeet during all weight bearing. He attends college and has minimal problems related to his hemophilia.

Surgical excision was utilized extensively after plasma concentrates became available in 1968. Primary surgical indications were the documented progression of major long bone lesions and proximity to a major weight-bearing joint. General principles of surgical intervention as discussed in Chapter 2 were followed. Curettage and bone grafting were uniformly successful in the seven cases in which surgery was performed. All the grafts were incorporated rapidly; preoperative range of motion was regained in adjacent joints; there has been no radiographic evidence of pseudotumor recurrence. Three postoperative complications occurred. Two wounds developed hematomas and healed by secondary intention. Deep sepsis did not occur. The single patient with Factor IX deficiency developed a large pulmonary embolus following curettage and grafting of a proximal tibial cyst. The usual treatment was followed and the patient recovered uneventfully.

MANAGEMENT

A pseudotumor of the small bones of the hands or feet is suspected when an area remains persistently swollen, occasionally erythematous, and tender in spite of adequate concentrate administration and rest. Radiographic confirmation is obtained. These small lesions are managed by a regimen of immobilization including well padded casting in the lower extremities, administration of concentrate to attain 50 percent factor levels for a ten day to two week minimal period, and diagnostic measures to determine the presence or absence of associated infection. Since these lesions are intracortical or even intramedullary in location, *aspiration should not be attempted.* Most of these small lesions will heal spontaneously with extended concentrate administration, rest, and time. Irradiation does not appear to materially alter their course. Long-term, protected weight bearing may decrease the amount of subsequent bony collapse.

Lesions of long bones and the bones of the pelvis can be extremely serious. When these lesions are symptomatic, progressing, or of a size or location to compromise joint function, they should be excised and bone grafted. Surgical management should follow the guidelines in Chapter 2. A persistent area of swelling in an extremity should always lead one to request a radiograph of the involved part.

Prompt infusion of clotting factors, when musculoskeletal bleeding occurs, has greatly reduced the frequency of large hematoma formation. Long bone fractures are managed as they are in nonhemophiliacs so that the incidence of nonunion, in the past frequently associated with pseudotumor formation, is markedly lowered. Most important, major surgical procedures can be performed with little increased risk or bleeding; thus, early and definitive treatment of pseudotumors is possible.

REFERENCES

1. Duthie, R. B., Matthews, J. M., Rizza, C. R., and Steel, W. M.: *The Management of Musculoskeletal Problems in the Haemophilias.* Blackwell Scientific Publications, Oxford, 1972.
2. Gunning, A. J., Biggs, R., and MacFarlane, R. G.: *Treatment of Hemophilia and Other Coagulation Disorders.* F. A. Davis Company, Philadelphia, 1966.
3. Gilbert, M. S.: Characterizing the hemophilic pseudotumor, in *Recent Advances in Hemophilia.* New York Academy of Sciences, New York, 1975.
4. Fernandez de Valderrama, J. A., and Matthews, J. M.: The haemophilic pseudotumor or haemophilic subperiosteal haematoma. J. Bone Joint Surg. 47-B, 1965.

9

GENERAL DENTAL MANAGEMENT

David Powell

The patient with hemophilia presents a challenge for the dentist to effectively and safely treat. A basic understanding of normal hemostasis as well as the physiology of the disorder are prerequisites for providing any dental care. Certain modifications in the dental techniques are made to assure safe treatment; however, quality dental care is not compromised. The hemophilic patient must enjoy all the advantages of quality restorative and preventive dentistry to maintain good oral health. Dental neglect, resulting in the need to remove nonrestorable teeth, presents serious management problems. Comprehensive care including semiannual examinations, proper oral hygiene, and patient/parent education, will minimize greatly the need for extractions and extensive dental restorations (Figs. 9-1 and 9-2).

Many hemophiliacs have neglected dental care for a number of reasons. Many persons with hemophilia, because of their frequent needs for medical care and hospitalizations, are crisis oriented. Since dental problems are not life threatening, the importance of regular dental care is not acknowledged; additionally, many dentists are unwilling or unable to provide treatment.

Recent hematologic advances have improved the clinical management of hemophilia. A dentist, with an understanding of these advances and a basic concept of the hematology of the disorder, can safely treat the hemophiliac. Contact between the dentist and the patient's hematologist and physician is imperative to ensure a safe course of treatment. Each patient's care and treatment plan must be evaluated on an individual basis after appropriate consultation as indicated.

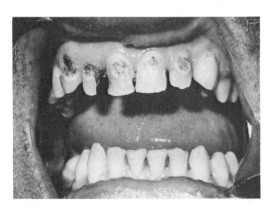

Figure 9-1. Gross caries in a 22-year-old severe classic hemophiliac who has neglected caring for his teeth. His dental problems could have been entirely prevented through proper and regular dental care.

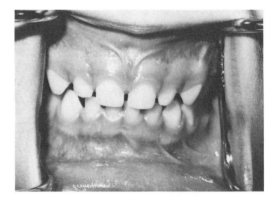

Figure 9-2. Excellent condition of a four-year-old child with severe hemophilia. Through proper care and a prevention program, he can be expected to have minimal dental problems.

EVALUATION

A complete history and a physical examination are essential prior to performing any dental treatment. The type and severity of hemophilia should be known; the history should include information about affected relatives and siblings, about plasma products which the patient has received, and whether he is on a home transfusion program. A general medical history is obtained to determine the presence of concurrent medical conditions which could influence the treatment plan. (Refer to Appendix 5 for form used for medical and dental history.) The dental history encompasses the type and outcome of previous dental treatment including extractions, as well as any complications with oral bleeding. The oral examination includes (1) extraoral findings: facial skin, salivary glands, temporomandibular joint, lips, etc.; (2) intraoral findings: tongue, throat, etc.; (3) periodontal findings; and (4) charting of the dental findings. The normal full mouth radiologic survey is taken. Care is exercised in the placement of the film to avoid producing a sublingual hematoma.

A treatment plan is developed and discussed with the patient and/or parent; consultation with the patient's physician and hematologist is indicated since medical management of the patient will be a cooperative effort.

PREVENTIVE MEASURES

Regular brushing, prophylaxis, and gingival massage will ultimately reduce decay and periodontal disease and decrease the tendency for gingival tissue to bleed secondary to abrasions from the toothbrush. A preventive program is adopted for all hemophilic patients since the difficulties and financial costs associated with restorative or surgical procedures mandate prevention of dental disease. All patients receive preventive dental education. The role of various foods in causing decay is explained; a balanced, sensible diet is encouraged with limited consumption of refined carbohydrates. When patients do consume "sweets," it is important that these be eaten with a meal prior to toothbrushing. Between-meal-snacks are most conducive to caries. Dietary analysis is important for those patients with a high DMF (decay, missing, filled) index. Parents of a hemophilic child are made aware of the importance of regular examinations and prophylaxis so that restorative and surgical problems are prevented.

Plaque Control

Toothbrushing must not be avoided due to fear of gingival bleeding. The slight hemorrhaging which may occur in the sulcus area is no more significant than for the nonhemophilic patient; good oral hygiene will reduce or eliminate this bleeding (Fig. 9-3). The hemophilic pa-

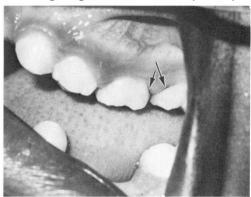

Figure 9-3. The arrows indicate very slight gingival oozing due to tooth brushing. This slight mucosal bleeding is no cause for alarm; good oral hygiene will minimize such bleeding.

tient uses a soft, multitufted toothbrush of an appropriate size. Brushing techniques are adapted to the patient's age, dexterity, and dentition. The techniques are similar to those used with other patients; exceptions include those patients younger than eight years of age who lack the dexterity required for most brushing methods. Those patients with motion limitations of the elbow, forearm, or wrist require special techniques. A toothpaste is preferred which contains fluoride and is pleasing to the child. Children should develop the habit of brushing following meals. The parent should examine the mouth and, when necessary, assist the child in a more acceptable performance. Disclosing agents, such as F.D.S. Red #3 (erythrosin), are useful in measuring tooth cleanliness. When these agents are applied to the teeth, the bacterial plaques become stained thus showing the parent and the child which areas are not properly brushed. A graphic means to check the oral hygiene technique is provided (Fig. 9-4).

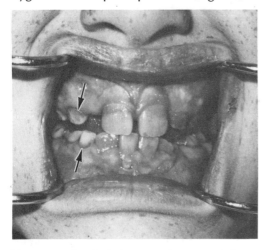

Figure 9-4. The disclosing agent has stained plaque (arrows) which remains on this child's teeth. The red stained plaque shows areas where tooth brushing is inadequate.

All patients are instructed in the use of dental tape or floss; dental tape is preferred because it causes less trauma to the tissue. When flossing is performed correctly, interproximal hemorrhage does not occur. The floss is "sawed" through the contact area; each approximating tooth surface is cleaned by vertical movement to avoid injury to the attached epithelium. Parents of children under age eight perform the flossing. Slight gingival bleeding caused by the flossing is not a reason for concern.

Systemic administration of fluoride is encouraged for those children age 12 and younger when they live in areas without fluoride in the water supply. Bottled fluoridated water and fluoride tablets, liquids, or vitamins are used systemically. A semiannual application of topical fluoride provides added resistance to tooth decay. In caries prone patients, top-

ical fluoride administered on a daily basis is beneficial.

Scaling and Polishing

All patients are on a six month recall program. Those patients with a high DMF index and poor hygiene are seen more frequently. At each recall the teeth are scaled and polished as indicated. Children have little, if any, calculus. If calculus is present, it is removed without undue trauma to the gingival tissue. Superficial bleeding resulting from careful scaling will cease within a reasonable period of time as will the slight hemorrhages which may occur with prophy cup polishing. Plasma products are adminis-

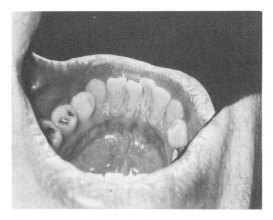

Figure 9-5. Supragingival calculus and stain on a 20-year-old severe hemophiliac who had never had his teeth cleaned.

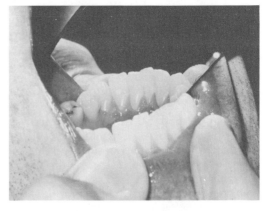

Figure 9-6. The same patient immediately after careful scaling and polishing without gingival bleeding and without prior replacement therapy.

tered prior to scaling when adult or teen-aged patients require deep scaling due to gross calculus. However, it may be possible to scale a quadrant at each dental appointment so that trauma is reduced and replacement therapy can be avoided (Figs. 9-5 and 9-6).

The determination to use replacement therapy is made on an individual basis with medical consultation. Factors to be considered are the severity of the hemophilia and the degree of anticipated trauma. When replacement therapy is used, the entire mouth is scaled at a single appointment so that the expense of blood products for subsequent appointments is avoided. Sufficient time is allowed at each appointment so that each procedure is performed with extra caution.

All calculus is removed with minimal trauma. Packing the sulcus with retraction cord is helpful to remove gross calculus because better access is obtained for instruments with lessening of tissue trauma. Use of the cavitron is not prohibited for removal of gross supragingival calculus; however, hand instruments are more appropriate for subgingival scaling so that tissue damage is reduced. Polishing the teeth requires additional caution so that bleeding caused by the rubber cup is superficial, minimal, and pressure controlled.

RESTORATIVE PROCEDURES

Restorative dentistry is performed in the usual manner. A rubber dam with a Young's frame is used to isolate the operating field. A lightweight rubber dam is used as there is less chance to torque the clamp which could abrade the gingiva. Additionally, the dam retracts the cheeks, lips, and tongue. Since these areas are highly vascular, their accidental laceration presents difficult management problems. Rubber dam clamps are selected and placed to minimize gingival trauma; wedges and matrices are used routinely and, with careful placement, do not produce significant bleeding. Crown preparation and placement present no

problems when the gingival portion of the tooth is carefully prepared and the crown is carefully fitted. Packing the tissues with gingival retraction cord is advantageous when extensive decay is evident. Crevice formation is avoided during the packing. When taking impressions, periphery wax is used on the tray to prevent possible intraoral laceration during tray placement (Fig. 9-7).

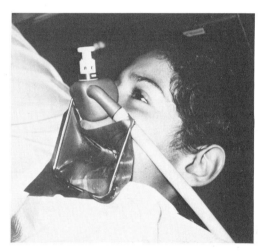

Figure 9-7. A ten-year-old patient with moderate hemophilia is prepared for restorative dentistry. He has received replacement therapy, has had block anesthesia, and has been given nitrous oxide to reduce his anxiety. The routinely used rubber dam protects the tongue and lips from accidental trauma.

High speed vacuum and saliva ejectors are used with caution so that sublingual hematomas are not created. Those ejectors with rubber padded tips are preferred since sublingual tissue cannot be drawn into the opening.

ANESTHETIC MANAGEMENT

The management and elimination of pain is one of the most difficult problems in providing dental care to the hemophilic patient. In the past, local anesthetics were not used since a dissecting hematoma with potential airway obstruction could result from local block anesthesia. Case histories were reported of death resulting from local anesthetics for dental procedures.

With the advent of plasma concentrates and cryoprecipitates, anesthetic and analgesic techniques were added to the realm of restorative procedures. The technique used is the most conservative method of pain control which is effective for the individual patient and for the procedure. A patient is not asked nor expected to endure painful procedures without relief. When this occurs, poor dental care will result and patients will return with great reluctance.

The following section outlines current anesthetic and analgesic techniques as well as the indications for each.

1. *No local anesthetic* is the method of choice when restoring primary teeth. Class I, II, III, IV, and V restorations are painlessly performed without local anesthesia. In the absence of an anesthetic agent, psychological preparation of the patient is important fortified with continuing verbal support. New, sharp burs are necessary and are used with very light pressure at high speed. Most procedures are performed on our pedodontic patients using this technique; however, the entire procedure is carefully explained to the child. He is reassured that anesthesia can be used if he feels discomfort. He is not allowed to "suffer through" the treatment.

Analgesia or anesthesia are used almost routinely for restorative or operative procedures on permanent teeth except for "pit" fillings which may not require anesthetics.

2. *Premedication analgesics* are used to raise the pain threshold or to relax the patient; however, this technique is not sufficient for very painful procedures. Nitrous oxide is a useful adjunct to reduce mild pain sensations.

3. *Pericemental injections,* although used in oral surgery, are not indicated for restorative dentistry because these injections do not produce the profound, long lasting anesthesia necessary for operative procedures. Additionally, these injections may produce a pressure ischemia resulting in a nonvital tooth.

4. *Infiltration and block anesthetics* are used only when the patient has received prior replacement therapy to elevate the plasma factor level to 50 percent. By attaining this 50 percent level, the few hours' time lag between infusion and the dental appointment are considered; thus, the dentist is assured that his patient has at least a 30 percent level during the dental procedures. The 50 percent levels are attained prior to the use of infiltration and block anesthetics since the injections are often deep into soft tissues and present greater potentials for problematic bleeding and its control. As noted in Chapter 10, 20 percent levels are sufficient for surgical procedures since bony areas are involved where better control of bleeding is possible; additionally, the injection is into more confined areas and not into deep soft tissues.

Mandibular blocks, posterosuperior blocks, and infiltration injections can be safely given. If the injection does not produce a bloody aspirate and no hematoma develops, further replacement therapy or other treatment is not indicated. However, with a bloody aspiration, careful surveillance is maintained for possible hematoma formation. If a hematoma develops, ice is applied to the area; the patient receives other infusions of plasma products with dosage and frequency at the discretion of the hematologist.

This approach contradicts most references appearing in the dental literature; however, many of these were prepared prior to the use of concentrates to manage the patient's hematologic defect. With preanesthetic administration of plasma products, over 200 blocks have been given safely without complications. Two positive aspirations were obtained but no hematomas have formed in this group of anesthetic blocks.

5. *Intrapulpal injections* are given safely for all pulpal procedures. Prior replacement therapy is unnecessary.

For all injections, a sharp 27 gauge needle is used. This size allows aspiration while minimizing tissue trauma. Slow injection of the solution, over a two minute period, further reduces tissue trauma.

An example of the clinical treatment record is found in Appendix 5.

PULPAL THERAPY

Pulpotomy, pulpectomy, and root canal fillings are preferable to extraction. Normally, when the pulp is necrotic, anesthetics are unnecessary. When vital pulp is exposed and anesthesia is required, the intrapulpal technique is the one of choice; it provides profound anesthesia without the need for infiltration, block injections, or prior replacement therapy.

Hemorrhage produced by pulp amputation or extirpation is controlled by pressure or a hemostatic agent such as epinephrine on a cotton pellet. If necessary to control hemorrhage, a pellet of formocresol is sealed in the pulp chamber for one week to mummify and fix the pulp tissue. Hemorrhage control during pulpal therapy is not a problem whether or not replacement therapy is utilized.

Root canal therapy is performed cautiously to avoid filing beyond the apex of the root; without caution, periapical bleeding occurs and is difficult to control. Therefore, canals are filed and filled slightly short, about 1 to 2 mm, of the radiographic apex.

ORTHODONTIC TREATMENT

Orthodontics to improve the well being and the appearance of the child should not be denied the hemophilic patient. The decision to perform orthodontia for the hemophiliac is made in a manner similar to that for other children. Considerations include the type of malocclusion, the esthetics, the function, and the desires of the parents and the child. The treatment is planned as it would be for any other patient without compromise. Improved occlusion will ultimately allow the maintenance of better oral hygiene, which will result in fewer dental and periodontal problems and a healthier oral mucosa.

Both interceptive (preventive) and full banded orthodontics are successfully performed. The choice of bicuspid extraction is determined by the individual case. Extraction, when indicated, is performed by the oral surgeon as an elective procedure.

Care must be taken in the adaptation and placement of bands and wires to avoid laceration of the oral mucosa; additional caution must be observed to avoid protruding sharp edges. Oral hygiene must be meticulous or the gingival tissue will become inflamed, edematous, and hemorrhagic from routine mastication and inadequate brushing. A Water Pik is essential in proper home care for the child with bands on his teeth.

EXFOLIATING PRIMARY TEETH

Loose, deciduous teeth occasionally pose a bleeding problem for a child since the tooth continuously traumatizes the tissue causing prolonged oozing. When this occurs, the tooth is extracted following infusion of appropriate plasma products. At the discretion of the hematologist or pediatrician, replacement therapy may continue after extraction. Epsilon-aminocaproic acid (EACA) is a treatment adjunct since it prevents premature lysis of the formed clot. The usual dosage for a child is 5 grams/day given in divided doses four times daily; the EACA is continued for seven days. It is available in liquid and tablet form. Emphasis is made that primary teeth are *not* routinely extracted prior to exfoliation; extraction is performed only when the sharp edges of the roots traumatize the gingiva and cause prolonged bleeding.

Other necessary extractions are performed with or by the oral surgeon. (Refer to Chapter 10 for a complete description of oral surgical management.)

CASE HISTORIES

Operative dentistry on the primary teeth of a severe hemophiliac with an inhibitor is illustrated by this case history.

J.G., four and one half-year-old boy with less than 1 percent Factor VIII and an inhibitor was initially seen in the dental clinic for evaluation of his dental status and treatment needs. His medical history was negative except for the hemophilia with an inhibitor. At this screening visit the dental program was explained to his mother; preventive dentistry was stressed including the importance of good oral hygiene, diet, and regular dental examinations.

Complete examination, roentgenograms, prophylaxis, and topical fluoride application were included at the next dental visit. Disto-occlusal decay of both mandibular primary molars (#S and #L) and extensive decay on the lower right second primary molar (#T) were revealed by clinical examination and confirmed on the radiographs. Dental prophylaxis with a rubber cup and prophy paste removed plaque; fluoride application followed. Replacement therapy was contraindicated because of the inhibitor presence. Additionally, painless restoration of the primary teeth was planned without local anesthesia.

At the operative visit, a 3A rubber dam clamp was carefully placed on tooth #T; a light weight rubber dam was positioned. A wedge, previously placed between tooth #S and #T, protected the papilla. The patient evidenced no distress during these procedures. A carious pulp exposure resulted from removal of decay from tooth #T. Intrapulpal anesthesia preceded the pulpotomy; pulpal bleeding was controlled by pressure. A pellet of formocresol was sealed in the pulp chamber and the tooth temporized with a zinc-oxide and eugenol cement. A disto-occlusal (DO) amalgam was placed in tooth #S. Routine wedges and matrices were used without compromise of cavity preparation.

At the subsequent visit, a DO amalgam was placed in a similar manner in tooth #L using a rubber dam. Following placement of the clamp and the rubber dam on tooth #T, the pulpotomy was completed and the tooth was prepared for a stainless steel crown. The gingival preparation was carefully managed. After the dam removal, the crown was carefully adapted and cemented; its margins were kept below the gingival tissue. Routine cleaning and polishing followed.

No bleeding or pain problems were experienced by the child during or after completion of the procedures. The importance of good routine dental care was re-emphasized to the mother because of the problems of anesthetic management with the presence of the inhibitor.

The second case history demonstrates extensive operative dentistry, using replacement therapy and local anesthesia.

D. H., a 17-year-old classic hemophiliac with a Factor VIII level of 2 percent, presented with a number of carious teeth, a malocclusion with anterior crowding, missing teeth, poor oral hygiene, and no restorations.

At the initial appointment, full mouth X-rays were taken and dental prophylaxis was performed using scalers to remove slight supragingival calculus. The teeth were then polished with a rubber cup and pumice paste. Carious teeth were present in all four quadrants while the mandibular right first molar (#30) had been extracted and the lower right third molar (#32) was congenitally missing. The maxillary right and left third molars (#1 and #16) and the mandibular left third molar (#17) were present but unerupted. The planned restorations and methods of anesthetic management were explained to the patient and parent. The importance of good hygiene was re-emphasized.

Arrangements were made for the patient to receive Factor VIII concentrate to attain plasma factor levels of 50 percent prior to each dental appointment when local anesthesia was anticipated.

At the next visit, left and right mandibular blocks were performed using 27 gauge needles, aspirating syringes, and 2 ml carpules of Xylocaine. Class I and Class II amalgams were placed in the mandibular right second molar and first and second bicuspids (#31, #29, #28) and mandibular left second molar and first bicuspid (#18, #21); due to the extensive decay, a stainless steel crown was placed on the lower left first molar (#19).

At the subsequent appointment, following infusion of plasma concentrate, right and left posterosuperior alveolar blocks were performed and amalgam fillings were placed in the maxillary right second molar (#2) and the maxillary left first and second molars (#14, #15). The maxillary right first molar (#3) with excessive decay, was restored with a stainless steel crown; amalgam restorations were placed in the maxillary right first and second bicuspids (#4, #5) and the maxillary left second bicuspid (#13). Lingual pit composite fillings were placed in the maxillary right and left lateral incisors (#7, #10) preceded by infiltration anesthesia in the appropriate areas. For all operative procedures, profound anesthesia was achieved without swelling or hematoma formation. The rubber dam, wedges, and matrices were used routinely. All preparations and procedures were not modified except to carefully avoid tissue trauma. After each appointment, the patient was cautioned to refrain from biting or chewing his anesthetized lip, tongue, or cheek. All restorations were polished at a later visit and fluoride applied to the teeth without prior concentrate administration. Measures to reduce plaque formation were re-emphasized to the patient. He expressed no interest in orthodontic treatment although he would benefit from it. He was placed on a regular six-month recall.

Extensive operative dentistry, root canal therapy, and a single extraction are described in this third case history.

W. D., age 47 with severe classical hemophilia, was referred to the dental clinic by the team oral surgeon because of many grossly carious teeth that hopefully could be restored (Fig. 9-8). In addition to hemophilia, he had moderately controlled diabetes. His past dental treatment included numerous extractions; two teeth had amalgam

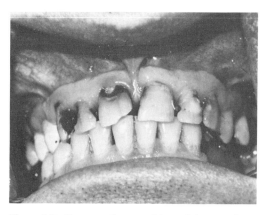

Figure 9-8. Preoperative condition of the mouth.

fillings. He desired salvage of as many teeth as possible.

At the first two appointments, full mouth radiographs were taken; an oral examination was done; the teeth were scaled and polished; and a treatment plan discussed. Although moderate calculus was present, plasma concentrate was unnecessary due to careful scaling. At the next two visits following decay

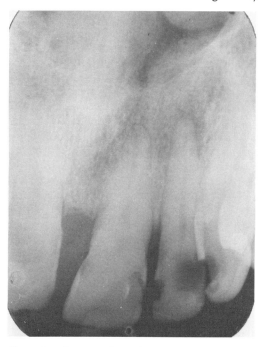

Figure 9-9. Preoperative radiograph shows extensive deep decay of the maxillary anterior teeth. The lateral incisor (#10) required root canal treatment as the pulp was nonvital.

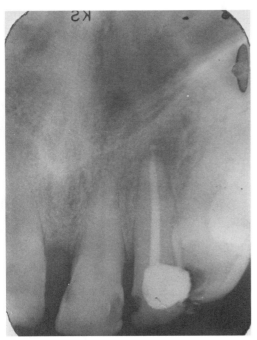

Figure 9-10. Postoperative radiograph shows the completed root canal. Care was taken to avoid filing beyond the apex since this could induce hemorrhage in an area where control may be difficult.

removal, endodontics were performed on the upper left lateral incisor (#10), a nonvital tooth (Fig. 9-9). The canal was filled with gutta-percha (Fig. 9-10).

Since the patient participated in the home transfusion program, he infused sufficient AHF concentrate to attain 50 percent levels prior to the next dental session. Because of the costs of concentrate, the remaining operative procedures were planned for one appointment even though many teeth were involved and the procedures were time consuming. A posterosuperior block provided anesthesia for the maxillary right second molar (#2) which required a Class II amalgam; infiltration injections preceded placement of Class II amalgams in the maxillary right and left first and second bicuspids (#4, #5, #12, and #13). Infiltration was used also to anesthetize the maxillary anterior teeth (#6, #7, #8, #9, #10, #11) for restoration. Pericemental injections anesthetized the lower right third molar (#32) for extraction. After extraction, the socket was packed with Surgicel coated with powdered bovine thrombin. The postsurgical regimen of epsilon-amino-caproic acid and dietary restriction was the same as that described in Chapter 10. The patient was dismissed with no swellings, hematomas, or oral oozing. The anesthesia was profound with complete elimination of pain; the postoperative period was uneventful without swellings, hematomas, or oral oozing. When the patient returned four weeks later to have his fillings polished, the extraction site was healed normally (Fig. 9-11). He was placed on a six month recall.

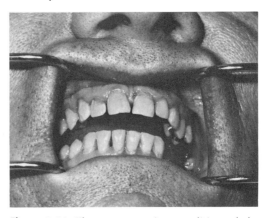

Figure 9-11. The postoperative condition of the mouth.

SUMMARY

Dental treatment represents a vital facet of the comprehensive care concept in treating persons with hemophilia. An enlightened dentist, with consultation from the appropriate medical personnel, can safely and effectively provide dental care which is painlessly delivered without compromise in quality. The basic principles of restorative dentistry are always observed although it may be occasionally necessary to modify operative techniques to treat the patient safely. Patient and parent education about the benefits of prevention are stressed since most dental problems can be eliminated or greatly reduced through a good prevention program. Due to the difficulties, risks, and expenses involved in providing restorative dentistry or oral surgery, it is imperative that the hemophiliac have regular dental examinations, prophylaxis, and fluoride treatments. Dentistry is one discipline where the hemophiliac can enjoy all the benefits of good health; prevention is the key.

REFERENCES

1. Steinle, C. J., and Kisker, C. T.: Pediatric dentistry for the child with hemophilia. N. Engl. J. Med. 283:1325–29, 1970.
2. Snyder, D. T., and Penner, J. A.: Preventive and restorative dental care for the hemophiliac. J. Mich. Dent. Assoc. 52:6–8, 1970.
3. Masterton, J. B.: Restorative dentistry for haemophiliacs. Br. Dent. J. 119:148–152, 1965.
4. Tichter, S., and Stratigos, G. T.: Management of a hemophiliac with a dental abscess and subsequent root canal therapy and apicoectomy. N.Y. State Dent. J. 39:11–14, 1973.
5. Nazif, M.: Local anesthesia for patients with hemophilia. J. Dentist. Child. 37:79–83, 1970.
6. Tarsitano, J., and Cohen, S.: Revelation and initial diagnosis of mild hemophilia from dental findings: report of case. J. Am. Dent. Assoc. 76:823–825, 1968.
7. Powell, D., and Bartle, J.: The hemophiliac: prevention is the key. Dent. Hygiene 48:214–219, 1974.

10

ORAL SURGICAL MANAGEMENT

Thomas F. Mulkey

EVALUATION

An important aspect of clinical care is the evaluation of the particular dental problem. Is surgical treatment necessary? Frequently, a patient with tooth pain expects extraction; however, after examination and X-ray, it is apparent that a filling or root canal therapy will save the tooth. Often, the cause of the pain is periodontal in origin and can be eliminated with proper professional care.

A consultation appointment, usually by referral from the staff of the Hemophilia Center or another dentist, is the initial contact with the hemophilic patient. A complete medical history is obtained as well as a determination of previous surgical procedures. Following a brief clinical examination of the mouth, radiographs are taken of all teeth in the upper and lower arches as well as views of the maxilla and mandible. After radiographic review and a more detailed examination of the mouth, the patient is advised of the necessary treatment. Surgical removal is indicated only after all conservative methods have been exhausted to attempt to save the tooth; extraction should then be accomplished quickly to relieve the patient's discomfort and anxiety.

Patient Preparation

The dental evaluation of a hemophilic patient for a surgical procedure must be thorough and complete. Because of their prior experiences with multiple hemorrhages and prolonged hospitalizations, adult patients, in particular, are normally very anxious and concerned about a possible surgical procedure. Therefore, time must be spent with the patient and his family to answer questions and to explain the planned surgery as well as the expected postsurgical events including those normal occurrences such as blood on the pressure dressing or the discolored stain found on the pillow the morning after the extraction. Each of these events can alarm the unprepared patient and his family. Since much of the success of dental surgical management of hemophilic patients depends upon the cooperation of the patient and his family, they must be aware of what is expected of them.

Medical Consultation

Consultation with the medical specialist—hematologist, pediatrician, or internist—in charge of the patient's medical care is essential. This specialist is responsible for determining the clotting deficiency and for establishing the type and dosage of plasma products needed to maintain hemostatic levels before and after surgery. Additionally, medical information can be supplied such as the presence of an inhibitor or other general medical problems which may alter the course of treatment. Background observations can also be furnished about the patient, i.e., how he reacts in stressful situations, how reliably he follows instructions. The oral surgeon informs the physician of the proposed treatment and exact techniques as well as the postoperative management; thus, possible postsurgical complications such as dehydration can be averted. The preoperative infusion therapy is planned; determination is made to treat the patient in or out of the hospital. Normally, surgeries are performed on an outpatient basis, however, if questions exist about the patient's ability to cooperate, he is not treated on an outpatient basis.

OPERATIVE PROCEDURES

Tooth extraction in a hemophilic patient should be as simple and as atraumatic as possible since the patient will have less anxiety about uncomplicated treatment. On the day of surgery the patient receives his presurgical infusion of the deficient factor at the Hemophilia Center or at home if he is on a self-transfusion program.[1] Then he reports to the oral surgery office accompanied by someone to drive him home. He has eaten nothing since midnight. Blood pressure and pulse recordings are made and an ultra-light barbiturate anesthesia is administered. The anesthetic is administered by the surgery-anesthesia team, described by Hubbell and Krugh[2] and further documented by Hagen and McCarthy.[3] The team is composed of the oral surgeon, the surgical assistant, and the anesthetic assistant; an endotracheal tube is not used.

The surgeon has training in all aspects of general anesthesia while the anesthetic assistant is practiced in the maintenance of a proper airway and in the monitoring of vital signs. Local anesthesia is used in all extraction procedures on hemophilic patients whether or not an ultra-light barbiturate anesthetic is utilized. The local anesthetic technique employs a 29 or 31 gauge needle, one half inch in length, and a carpule syringe (Fig. 10-1). The needle is positioned in the periodontal membrane space with the bevel against the tooth and the solution is injected with considerable difficulty. If the plunger is easily compressed, the needle is in the wrong position; it should be removed and reinserted. This injection technique is repeated in all four quadrants of the tooth: mesial, distal, buccal, and lingual. This technique is appropriate for single and multiple rooted teeth. No waiting period is required for anesthetic effect. After the last axial surface has been injected, the tooth may be removed. Unlike the usual local anesthetic techniques of infiltration or nerve block, this method is also effective when there is infection around the tooth.

It is unnecessary and undesirable to elevate a mucoperiosteal flap during tooth removal. The interdental papillae is incised; the tooth is luxated with a straight elevator and removed with a forcep. Any loose or sharp bone from alveolus fracture is removed. Following the extraction, a piece of Surgicel* dusted with topical powdered Bovine Thrombin†

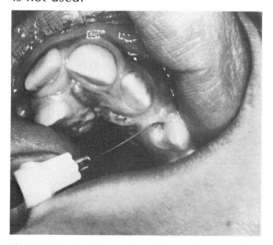

Figure 10-1. Needle positioned for pericemental injection.

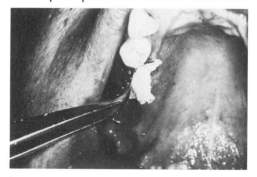

Figure 10-2. Surgicel placed in extraction socket.

*Surgical Absorbable Hemostat (oxidized regenerated cellulose), Johnson and Johnson.

†Thrombin, Topical, (bovine origin), Parke Davis.

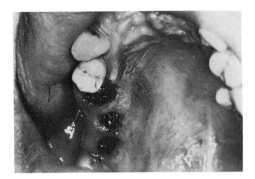

Figure 10-3. Extraction sites immediately following Surgicel placement.

is placed in the apical portion of each root socket (Figs. 10-2 and 10-3). A 4 inch by 4 inch gauze pressure dressing is placed over the extraction site; the ultra-light barbiturate anesthesia is discontinued. Anesthetic recovery occurs in 10 to 15 minutes in the average case.

POSTSURGICAL MANAGEMENT

The pressure dressing remains intact for eight hours following the surgery. Immediately upon postanesthetic recovery, epsilon-amino-caproic acid (EACA) is administered. The initial dosage is 5 gm; subsequent dosages are 2.5 gm every six hours for ten days.

The postextraction diet control is vital and is enforced for a 10 day period. For 24 hours, the patient ingests nothing except the EACA and sufficient water to swallow any other necessary medication. After the initial 24 hour period and continuing for the next 48 hours, he may consume unlimited quantities of cool, clear liquids excluding milk and other dairy products. These items are restricted because they deposit sediment and a film residue which may lead to early clot degeneration. A straw is not allowed since the sucking action may dislodge a clot; for the same reason, the liquids must be swallowed immediately and not retained in the mouth. A pureed diet is consumed on the fourth postextraction day. Thus, the patient can eat any food item which does not require chewing. Use of a blender permits a varied diet with complete nutrition. The pureed diet continues for seven days at which time the patient gradually resumes his regular diet.

The extraction site is not sutured nor is it protected with any type of surgical splint. During the eight hours postsurgically, the only protection given the clot is from the gauze pressure dressing. After this period, the clot is preserved by dietary control and the use of EACA. As the healing progresses, the clot appears to "grow" out of the socket.

During the first postextraction day, the clot is larger but appears much as it did immediately following surgery (Fig. 10-4). By the third day it has enlarged, become smooth and shiny in appearance, and may have partially retracted (Fig. 10-5). By the seventh postsurgical day, the clot has retracted with sloughing of the overabundant mass; the socket has become visible with a healthy fibrin covered clot now apparent (Fig. 10-6).

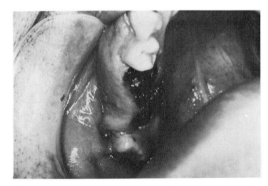

Figure 10-4. Extraction sites on first postoperative day.

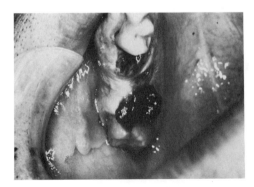

Figure 10-5. Extraction sites on third postoperative day.

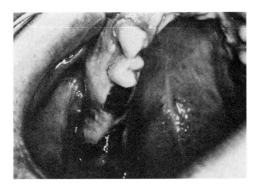

Figure 10-6. Sites on seventh postoperative day.

Adjunctive Medication

The use of medications in the treatment of hemophiliacs for tooth extraction must include the infusion of the deficient factor to attain 20 percent clotting factor levels prior to the extraction. The use of plasma products following the surgery is instituted if any bleeding occurs; then the deficient factor level is elevated to 30 to 50 percent. When bleeding occurs and plasma products are required, dietary control returns to the cool, clear liquid stage.

As previously noted, epsilon-amino-caproic acid is always used to inhibit the plasminogen activation and to prevent clot lysis. EACA has proven extremely useful to prevent postextraction bleeding without subsequent infusions of the deficient factor.[4] A 10 day regimen with administration every six hours around the clock is the most effective. Antibiotics and pain medication are used as necessary in the preoperative or postoperative period. As mentioned in Chapters 2 and 3 the use of aspirin is discouraged. Oral medications, taken the first postoperative day, are swallowed with a minimum amount of water. The use of other routine medications is supervised by the patient's physician.

OUTPATIENT CONCEPT

Outpatient dental extractions have been carried out at the Hemophilia Rehabilitation Center since August 1966. With additional experience it became apparent that most hemophilic patients were capable of the complete cooperation necessary for successful outpatient management. From 1966 through 1973, 361 outpatient extractions have been performed; during the same period 167 extractions have been managed in the hospital.

Daily contact is established with the patient during the 10 day postextraction period. Either the telephone or an in-person interview are used to determine the patient's status, to answer his questions, to reassure him, and to reinforce the necessary dietary control. He is reminded to administer his EACA at the six hour intervals. This daily follow-up provides a necessary check and balance for outpatient management and also gives a sense of security to the patient. The historic concept of inpatient treatment of hemophiliacs is well entrenched in the minds of many physicians; however, it is not desirable for the patient to be separated from his family during a stressful period if hospitalization is not really necessary. For the emotional security of the patient it is essential to assure him that he can be admitted to the hospital if this should become necessary. Many patients, previously treated on an inpatient basis, become quite apprehensive at the prospect of outpatient care. On the second occasion for surgery, the same individual appears less anxious about the out-of-hospital management.

Another major factor in the consideration of outpatient versus inpatient care is the cost of the latter. The total cost of extraction of several teeth becomes significant when the expense of the plasma products is coupled with the costs of several days' hospitalization. The capacity to eliminate the in-hospital costs permits a marked reduction in expenses. A further reduction in the cost of dental care could be made if the patient and his family were better educated in the preventive aspects of dental care; then emergency measures would be unnecessary.

SPECIAL PROBLEMS

Multiple Extractions

Ordinarily, in our outpatient surgery the number of extracted teeth is limited to four anterior and two posterior teeth since sutures or splints are not routinely used and it is important to limit the number of bleeding sockets. However, if more teeth must be extracted and possibly the mouth prepared for dentures with alveolectomies, sutures are used. At the time of suture removal, it has *not* been necessary to raise the deficient clotting factor level to obtain hemostasis. Hospitalization is not necessary if plasma products are available on an outpatient basis.

The following case history describes the complete edentulation, with six different surgical procedures, of a mild hemophiliac:

This 50-year-old man with Factor VIII levels of 19 percent was first seen in 1969 with complaints of pain and discomfort in the maxillary right central incisor. Radiographs revealed advanced periodontal disease throughout the mouth. Only 13 of his permanent teeth were present; the multiple missing teeth had been replaced by maxillary and mandibular partial dentures. Typical of most hemophiliacs, whose previous extractions occurred before concentrate was available, he wanted only the one offending tooth removed. After the infusion of 400 units of Factor VIII concentrate, the tooth was removed atraumatically. The patient followed the postsurgical routine and had no bleeding; further Factor VIII infusions were unnecessary. The lack of postsurgical complications was almost unbelievable to this patient since his previous extractions had been difficult. Eleven months later, the maxillary left lateral incisor and mandibular left third molar were extracted following infusion of 400 Factor VIII units. Again, postextraction bleeding was absent. On subsequent visits, over a three year period, two or

three teeth were removed; postextraction hemorrhage never occurred. The patient was fitted with maxillary and mandibular dentures following complete edentulation. To summarize, during 6 office visits, 13 teeth were removed from this mild hemophiliac. The total costs of the edentulation including the replacement therapy were approximately $500.00. The patient lost no time from work except the one half day per visit for the infusion and extraction. He was spared the emotional trauma of separation from his family. If all the extractions had been performed in the hospital at one time under general endotracheal anesthesia, a minimum of three to five hospital days would have been required. The total Factor VIII consumption would have been much greater due to the increased number of potential bleeding sites. The total costs for in-hospital care would have ranged from $1000 to $1800. He would have been absent from work five to seven days and he would have been separated from his family during a period of stress.

Pseudotumors

Pseudotumors of the mandible and maxilla are rare. Three cases have been encountered at this Center. The first case occurred in the right mandibular first

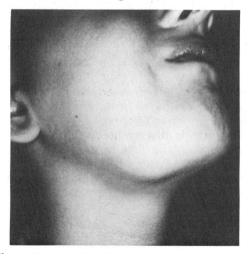

Figure 10-7. Hard swelling in right submandibular region.

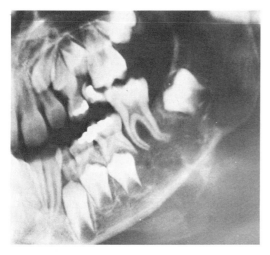

Figure 10-8. Lateral jaw radiograph showing inferior bony expansion, hypereruption of the mandibular first molar, and the osteolytic nature of the lesion.

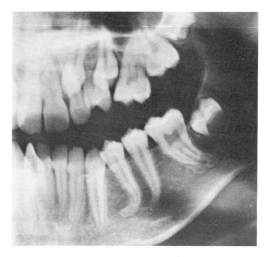

Figure 10-10. Four year postcurettage radiographs show complete healing of osteolytic lesion with normal development and eruption of permanent teeth.

molar region of an eight-year-old boy (Figs. 10-7 and 10-8). The tumor expanded the angle of the mandible with a resultant elevation of the tooth from the socket. The tooth was extracted and the vascular lesion was curetted; Factor VIII concentrate was administered for nine days to maintain 50 percent levels. No recurrence was evident during the following four years; functional recontouring of the skeletal deformity occurred (Figs. 10-9 and 10-10).

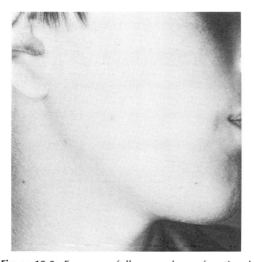

Figure 10-9. Four year follow-up shows functional recontouring of the right mandible.

The second lesion was in the mandible of a seven-year-old boy. Treatment was similar to that described in the previous paragraph. Unfortunately, the patient was lost to follow-up; subsequently he succumbed from a cerebral hemorrhage which occurred two years after the pseudotumor treatment.

The third case involved a 16-year-old patient who developed a swelling in the right mandible extending from the second bicuspid to the area of the coronoid notch. The lateral surface of the mandible had expanded; the lateral cortical plate had eroded and the soft tissues of the buccal pouch were involved. The mandibular right first and second molars were extracted and the area was curetted. This was performed in the hospital after infusion of Factor VIII concentrate twice daily to maintain his levels at 50 percent. Healing progressed uneventfully until nine months later when a recurrence of the tumor was evident. Again, after raising the Factor VIII level to 50 percent, the area was recuretted and two maxillary teeth, which had hypererupted into the soft tissue, were extracted. The lesion, now two years postcurettage, has nearly resolved; functional recontouring of the mandible is continuing.

Within the scope of our experience,

mandibular lesions have not been irradiated. Since developing tooth germs were present in the young patients just described, irradiation was not considered.

Patients with Inhibitors

These patients present special problems to the oral surgeons. The presence of a circulating anticoagulant eliminates the use of the concentrated plasma products. When an acute dental infection is present and is demanding intervention, antibiotic medication is instituted. The patient is hospitalized; epsilon-amino-caproic acid (EACA) is administered for 24 hours pre-extraction. The tooth is extracted using the previously described surgical procedure without suture or splints. The diet and EACA administration are rigidly controlled for the 10 day postsurgical period. In the case of nonsuppurative teeth, outpatient management is utilized with dietary control and EACA administration. Postsurgical bleeding responds to pressure and healing is uneventful.

Once a circulating anticoagulant is diagnosed, a program of parent and patient education is essential to attempt to prevent dental problems. When extraction is necessary, EACA administration, diet control, careful extraction with the special anesthetic techniques, and postsurgical follow-up care are essential.

SUMMARY

Any surgical procedure for the hemophiliac patient requires a thorough evaluation of the patient, consultation with his physician, and preparation of the patient and his family. Using the pericemental injection technique with local anesthesia, atraumatic extraction, and the described postextraction management of the socket, most hemophilic patients can be treated on an outpatient basis. A pretreatment evaluation and consultation visit is necessary to insure that the patient will accept and will cooperate with treatment. Postsurgical management requires strict dietary control and the judicious administration of epsilon-amino-caproic acid at 6 hour intervals for a 10 day period.

Special surgical problems are presented by those patients with a circulating anticoagulant, those needing multiple extractions, and those requiring any extensive soft tissue or intraosseous surgery. Ordinarily these special situations can be managed more satisfactorily in the hospital.

REFERENCES

1. Dietrich, S. L.: Modern management of hemophilia. J. School Health 43(2):81–83, 1973.

2. Hubbell, A. O., and Krugh, H. W.: Management of intravenous anesthesia to control recovery time. J. Oral Surg. Oral Med., Oral Pathol. 9:403–410, 1956.

3. Hagen, J. O., and McCarthy, F. M.: General anesthesia for the ambulatory patient: The anesthetic team. J. S. Calif. Dent. Assoc. 37:244–247, 1969.

4. Walsh, P. M., Rizza, C. R., Matthews, J. M., Eipe, J., Kernoff, P. B. A., Cole, M. D., Bloom, A. L., Kaufman, B. M., Beck, P., Hahan, C. M., and Biggs, R.: Epsilon-amino-caproic acid therapy for dental extractions in haemophilia and Christmas disease, a double blind controlled trial. Br. J. Haemotol. 20:463, 1971.

11

PSYCHOLOGICAL AND SOCIAL ASPECTS

Charles H. Hurt

OVERVIEW OF PSYCHOLOGICAL PROBLEMS OF HEMOPHILIC PATIENTS AND FAMILY MEMBERS

The diagnosis of hemophilia, usually confirmed in the child's first year of life, *always* creates stresses upon the family unit and all its members, particularly upon the mother, the father, and the affected child, but also upon siblings and the extended family. Whether the patient and/or the family members develop psychological problems attributable to these stresses depends upon the following factors: (1) the quality of their individual and combined emotional strengths, ego gratifications, and capacities for coping with stress; (2) the quality of medical care available, the promptness in securing treatment, and the adequacy of communication between health care personnel and the family; (3) the availability of quality educational and vocational opportunities; and (4) the utilization of preventive mental hygiene measures when needed.

Health care personnel who understand the psychological stresses upon family members may help to prevent the physical and emotional damage which sometimes results from hemophilia. Education and counseling of family members at the *earliest possible time* is extremely important. This counseling is a difficult task and its handling may set the tone for the long-term relationship with the family and the child.

There are no patterns of psychological problems which are characteristic of all hemophiliacs or their families, nor is it possible to identify a "hemophilic person-

ality." The range of problems encountered is extremely broad and extends from those evidenced by relatively stable individuals and families to those found in persons and families with severe degrees of personal and social disorganization. If the previously mentioned factors are not optimal, the child or adult with hemophilia may show some of these psychological manifestations: (1) *A low self-esteem and limited self-confidence* leading to excessive dependency and a failure to meet educational and vocational challenges; (2) *a delay in masculine identification* with resultant problems in male-female peer relations; (3) *a failure to accept the realities of hemophilia* leading to physical neglect, excessive use of drugs, severe crippling, or death; and (4) *a general prolonged immaturity* with rebellion to authority, and participation in "risk-taking" behavior which may represent a counterphobic response to anxiety.

Great care must be exercised in identifying risk-taking behavior. Most individuals with hemophilia assume moderate risks of injury at every stage of development through engaging in those activities important to their own physical and emotional development. Consequently, engaging in activities such as motorbike riding and skiing should not necessarily be viewed out of context as neurotic behavior.

If the psychological and social stresses which contribute to the previously mentioned manifestations are recognized and treated in childhood, their crippling consequences should not occur in adulthood. Just as prompt factor replacement therapy and exercise can minimize or prevent joint deformity, so can early counseling or psychotherapy with hemophilic boys and their parents minimize or prevent emotional handicaps. The etiology of psychological problems may be more clearly understood if we view some of the stresses experienced by the patient, his parents, and other family members.

Psychological Stresses on the Mother

Because the hemophilic boy's earliest and closest relationship is usually with his mother, an understanding and alleviation of her psychological stresses is of utmost importance. Whether or not these stresses create psychological problems for the mother depends upon her emotional strengths and personal gratifications, upon the supportive parental role assumed by the father, and upon the absence of serious reality problems such as severe poverty or the absence of adequate medical care. The most frequently observed problem is her tendency to overprotect and to place undue restrictions upon the child's activity and decision making because of her fear and anxiety about his possible injury or death. Her excessive anxiety may derive from prior experiences with a hemophilic brother, father, or uncle who suffered severe crippling and perhaps death in the absence of modern day treatment. For example, in her effort to protect her son, she may restrict him from engaging in normal recreational activities or from playing with other boys, she may enroll him in a school for the handicapped rather than in regular school, or she may perform for him many day to day tasks which he can manage himself. Under such circumstances the child remains dependent and infantile and is prevented from coping with the ordinary hazards and responsibilities of everyday life. In adolescence he may take unreasonable risks in a continuing rebellion to restraints or as an overcompensation for his fears. Or he may remain passive and dependent, experiencing conflict and delay in accepting adult responsibilities.

The mother may experience suppressed feelings of hostility, resentment, and antagonism toward her hemophilic son resulting from displaced feelings toward the hemophilic father or brother whose needs took precedence over her own in childhood. Since she contributed the defective gene to her son, the mother may feel guilty that she "caused" his disability; thus, she may become overly solicitous, indulgent, permissive, and experience difficulty in effecting discipline. Guilt feelings may be intensified if she knew prior to conception that she was a probable or obligatory carrier. She may feel that she failed because she did not produce a "normal, healthy son." If the boy's father considers her negligent and holds her responsible because hemorrhages occurred during his absence, she may feel guilt or anger. These feelings are intensified if, in fact, she *is* always responsible for securing appropriate and timely treatment.

She may be overburdened by her constant responsibility for accurately assessing the child's daily health status, for determining his need for treatment, and for establishing his activity level. These burdens are particularly troublesome if she has been unable to share this responsibility with the father or with the hemophilic boy. Problems are intensified by medical care and advice which is faulty, inconsistent, or poorly communicated resulting in confusion, indecision, or resistance to following the recommendations regarding the care of the child.

The mother's inability to provide adequate affection and care for her hemophilic child may also be linked to various other factors: insufficient gratification or instability in her current life situation, emotional deprivation in her own childhood, or her limited intellectual ability to understand medical advice and to make independent judgements.

Psychological Stresses on the Father

The role assumed by the father is the most important single factor in determining the hemophilic boy's satisfactory emotional adjustment. Since the mother may tend to overprotect her hemophilic son, he has an even greater need to identify with a masculine model. When the father extends himself to the hemophilic boy in a supportive, companionable manner during early childhood, the boy's emotional and social adjustment is likely to be satisfactory, despite the mother's tendency toward overprotection. The case of Kenny illustrates the importance of this relationship with the father:

Kenny G., the middle of three boys, was aged 12½ years when first seen at the Center for evaluation and treatment of a chronic knee flexion contracture which had resulted from a severe knee hemorrhage five years previously. Adequate orthopedic care had not been available in his small community and, having completed only a part of the first grade in regular public school at the time, Kenny was assigned a home teacher and remained out of school until the sixth grade. Although he spent most of this five year period in a wheelchair, his father had gone to great lengths to include Kenny in the activities enjoyed by the normal older and younger brothers. Fishing, hunting, mechanics, and other shared interests allowed Kenny to develop a strong identification with his father. Mr. G and the boys built models, raced miniature cars, and went riding together in the nearby hills on his father's motor bike. Kenny noted with pride: "Dad and I sure have to do some fast talking with Mother to get to do fun things."

Intensive physical therapy resulted in full knee extension and the capacity to walk, but school personnel and parents were apprehensive about Kenny's return to regular school. Despite their marked anxiety, both parents wanted him to attend public school; and they were able to resolve much of their conflict in 12 conjoint casework treatment hours, scheduled weekly, with an equal number of sessions for Kenny. The mother discussed at length her long standing fear for Kenny's safety

and her overprotection of him. She described heretofore unresolved feelings of grief following the death of their first child (nonhemophilic) at age 20 months, which she associated with her constant fear of losing Kenny. As she gained some understanding of her conflict in allowing him more freedom, with on-going emotional support from the father, Mrs. G. was able to allow Kenny to assume responsibility for selection of many of his own activities and to re-enter public school. Kenny made effective use of his own supportive sessions and was able for the first time to express fully to his mother his feelings about her overprotection, and to feel satisfaction in proving to her his own abilities to assume responsibility. He commented: "Mother holds on to me too much and is still afraid sometimes when I go out, but she'll get used to it." At the time of my most recent contact with him, Kenny was employed part-time, played tennis three times weekly, and attended college with the anticipation of studying law.

Thus, the father's participation in activities with the child and in his care helps to reduce the mother's feelings of guilt and her burden of responsibility. The boy finds it easier to cope with the mother's overprotection; he perceives his father's approval and he develops confidence that he can meet the father's expectations. In this process, he develops a sense of personal and physical adequacy. He realizes that his father expects him to assume responsibility for selecting safe and appropriate activities, and to move safely toward independence and separation from the mother. Consequently, the stresses on the father should be understood and alleviated at the earliest opportunity so that the boy can utilize these strengths from their relationship.

The father may experience feelings of rejection, anger, and frustration in relating to his son because of the latter's overdependence upon the mother. An excessively close, mutually satisfying relationship between the hemophilic boy and the mother may exclude the father, leaving him envious or threatened. A personally insecure father may regard his son as a fragile, imperfect extension of himself; he may be condescending toward the boy or withdraw from him. Usually, the mother transports the boy for treatment, examination, and consultation with Center staff. Thus, the father may lack important information about hemophilia and may fail to utilize the help of the professional staff to alleviate his fears and anxiety. Furthermore, if medical care insurance is inadequate or public supplemental assistance unavailable, the tremendous financial costs of treatment may become so burdensome and difficult to manage that the father experiences tension and negative feelings toward his hemophilic son. As with the mother, the father may also be unable to give affection and care to his hemophilic child because of his limited intellectual ability, insufficient life gratifications, or childhood emotional deprivation.

Psychological Stresses on the Patient

Compounded by often unresolved psychological stresses in his parental relationships, the maturing individual with hemophilia is confronted by multiple psychological and social stresses. From an early age, he experiences frustration from necessary restrictions and treatment procedures. He is expected to cope with the untimely occurrence of painful hemorrhages which result in immobilization, disruption of activities, hospitalization, and severe disability. Early in life, he begins to interrelate his experiences with the cause and effect of hemorrhages and, ideally, he begins to assume early independent responsibility for his physical activity and well-being. He is expected to avoid hazardous endeavors and to inform his parents promptly when hemorrhages occur, in spite of the possibility of tension and adverse parental feelings about the financial costs and inconvenience of securing treatment. He is expected to balance his tendencies toward impulsiveness and his wishes for independence, on the one hand, with parental anxiety and medical advice on the other. Despite the frustrations and disappointments of frequently disrupted educational and vocational plans, he is pressured to develop independent motivation toward appropriate life goals.

In early adulthood, he is expected to decide whether he will attempt to finance the high cost of his treatment through employment or whether he will become dependent upon private or governmental financial assistance. Often, these heavy expectations create apprehension and anxiety in the parents and the child, particularly if they have not made significant progress in coping with the realities of hemophilia during childhood.

Psychological Stresses on Other Family Members

If the parents of the hemophilic child fail to recognize and to fulfill the respective personal needs of their other children, these brothers and sisters of the affected boy may experience frustration and emotional deprivation in their own development. They may feel unloved, resentful, or envious of the extra parental attention, favoritism, or overprotection accorded to him; in turn, they may relate to him in neurotic ways. Thus, he may be unable to benefit from the normal give and take experiences of family life and may remain isolated or immature in his expectations of others.

The carrier daughter or the sister of the hemophilic may experience unnecessary stress about the certainty, or the possibility, that she is a carrier. She may have received inadequate information and preparation to help her solve her questions about child bearing. Her parents may have avoided this reality during her development because of their own unresolved conflicts about, or their unawareness of, the genetic aspects of hemophilia.

Grandparents or other members of the extended family may experience some of the same stresses felt by the parents. With fewer opportunities to resolve their apprehensions, these family members may respond to the child in ways that interfere with his normal development such as extreme overprotection. This situation can be controlled when the boy's parents, secure in their own respective roles, can interpret effectively his condition, abilities, and needs to members of the extended family. Brief professional counseling with members of the extended family may be helpful in resolving these problems as they arise.

PSYCHOLOGICAL TREATMENT AND PREVENTIVE MEASURES

The satisfactory psychological and social adjustment of the individual with hemophilia depends upon the successful resolution of the previously identified stresses affecting his parental relationships and his early emotional development. Many important personality features are established in the first six years of a child's life. The importance of this early growth period has long been recognized by behavioral scientists in their clinical observation of the personality development of normal individuals as well as of those who are emotionally disturbed. Comprehensive management of hemophilia must provide adequate medical care to minimize the occurrence of physical disabilities. It must also provide early prophylactic mental hygiene counseling, psychotherapy, and educational and vocational counseling as needed for the prevention of psychosocial disabilities.

Psychosocial Services

Diagnosis and treatment of psychological and social problems can be managed most effectively by the collaboration of a psychiatric social worker, a psychiatrist, a psychologist, and a rehabilitation counselor. These professionals should be available, even on a part time basis, through a Center providing the basic care for hemophilia. One or more of them should be qualified to do psychotherapy. As a member of a multidisciplinary staff, the psychotherapist can become aware of

all aspects of the disease; additionally, he can acquire valuable longitudinal knowledge of each patient and his family. When psychotherapy is unavailable at a Hemophilia Center, the professional staff of a community psychiatric facility or other agency may provide care. Information about hemophilia provided by the Center staff will facilitate the individual's use of these resources.

The psychiatric social worker on the staff of this Center is responsible for the diagnosis of psychological and social problems associated with hemophilia, and for the provision of individual and family psychotherapy to both children and adults. Consultation about specific patients is provided to other Center staff members and to hospital personnel as well as to school personnel and community agencies. Ready accessibility of the social worker to the hemophilia treatment room and to outpatient clinics provides the opportunity to observe manifestations of problems and to initiate timely referrals for treatment.

Psychological Treatment

Psychotherapeutic techniques and approaches are the same as those utilized for other individuals and families with emotional problems. However, the psychotherapist should be aware of the unique stresses of hemophilia upon various family members and should be sufficiently flexible to provide treatment or consultation when needed. Frequently, several members of the multidisciplinary team may be working simultaneously with the patient as was true in the case of Reuben.

Reuben M. was the younger child in a Mexican-American Catholic family which included his parents and an older sister who was married and in her own home before he was 16 years old. The occurrence of Reuben's severe hemophilia A was not surprising to the parents because two of his mother's brothers had died at ages five and three years following "internal bleeding" and head injury. Two of *her* maternal uncles with hemophilia had died before the age of 40. Consequently, she was exceedingly anxious and overprotective in her care of Reuben who was himself in his early 20s before the advent of plasma concentrates, home infusion program, and informed orthopedic management.

The parents' marriage was characterized by stability and mutual gratification and while Mrs. M. referred to her husband with affection and respect, she clearly regarded decisions concerning Reuben as being *her* primary responsibility and not her husband's. Characteristically, the father was a quiet, passive man who generally deferred to the mother's influence on matters concerning the boy. Reuben, who never directly expressed anger or differences of opinion to his father, commented: "I jumped when he was around." Occasionally, the father would insist upon letting Reuben try a new activity, but there were few companionable, masculine shared activities between them. Although Reuben worked for a short time in his father's auto repair shop he disliked the "dirt and grease" aspects of the job and soon quit. His mother placed a high value on Reuben's good manners, his overall conformity to her wishes, and his sensitivity to the feelings of others. Consciously, she would strive to allow Reuben a "normal childhood," but characteristically she discouraged his physical activities and his assertion of independence and doubted that he would ever be able to function independently. He did well in parochial school, but felt resentment and embarrassment because the school personnel insisted that his mother bring his lunch to him each day so that she could observe him during the noon recess.

Reuben, first seen for psychological evaluation at age 23, was living in his parents' home and had made only tentative and abortive gestures toward employment and separation from his parents. He was extremely cautious, po-

lite, self-effacing, and passive and expressed reservation about any decision which might not coincide with his mother's wishes. During the course of 20 weeks of psychotherapy, he became more able to express resentment about the necessity to secure his mother's permission to leave the house or to make even minor decisions. He described her "mother-knows-best" attitude and his frustration in not openly challenging her. He compared his current situation with early childhood memories when he regarded himself as "a puny little guy sitting at home, watching the world go by." He was aware that his parents saw him as being "weak and delicate," and that they never took his ideas very seriously.

Brief-term psychotherapy was focused in three major areas: (1) his ambivalence and conflicts about changing his passive-dependent relationship with his mother; (2) his low self-esteem, feelings of impotence, and struggles in role identification, which were intensified by pressure from a girlfriend toward independence, and (3) his doubts and insecurity about achieving vocational independence. With support, he was able to identify some of his own needs, to express his anger toward his mother, and to become more assertive with her. Concurrently, his mother was seen in several sessions for support and reassurance. Close collaboration was maintained with the vocational rehabilitation counselor who provided Reuben with emotional support and step by step assistance in securing training and employment. Concurrently, members of the orthopedic and hematology staff assisted Reuben by recommending assistive devices, exercise, and a self-transfusion program, which allowed him to administer plasma concentrate at home or at work. Shortly after the termination of counseling, Reuben was employed in the profession of medical photography and photomicroscopy. Subsequently, he was happily married to the girlfriend who was instrumental in encouraging his independence.

While group therapy may be efficacious for patients or parents, travel to a metropolitan center for regular group sessions may present a serious time problem for the patient or the parent especially when this commitment is added to other necessary clinical appointments. Relatively brief-term counseling or psychotherapy with individuals and/or family members suffices generally, particularly when treatment is not long delayed.

Ordinarily the availability of psychotherapy is more limited than the demands for this service; hence, careful selection is necessary to serve those individuals who are most able to utilize the treatment. Otherwise, inordinate amounts of time can be expended on persons who are poorly motivated or unable to benefit from psychotherapy. The popular fantasy persists that any individual who manifests distressing symptoms of social or psychological "maladjustment," or who prefers a life style radically different from one's own, can or should change as the result of psychotherapeutic intervention. Despite their unsuitability for psychotherapy, such individuals need to be seen because they do present symptoms which are most persistent or very distressing to family members or to Center staff; meanwhile, other patients or family members who might benefit from brief-term psychotherapy are deprived of this help. Consequently, Center staff conferences may be designed to spend time profitably considering the individual's motivation for change, his right to be a part of the decision for change, and the limits to which the institution and its personnel can extend themselves to meet his needs. Counseling with patients or their relatives may occasionally be accomplished more effectively by a team member other than the one usually responsible for the treatment of psychological problems. Good mental health should be the active concern of every team member.

Although psychological and social development of the hemophilic individual may appear to be unsatisfactory at various stages of life such as entry into school, adolescence, adulthood, marriage, and employment, delayed maturation and *not* specific psychosocial pathology may be responsible for this impression. Brief-term supportive counseling for the patient and the family members is of crucial importance at these stages. While a great majority of patients and their families function within normal limits in spite of the complications imposed by the disease, a small percentage require long-term psychotherapy. A still smaller percentage may require intensive inpatient psychiatric care.

The young adult's decision to depend upon a public assistance program providing subsistence and payment for medical care, rather than to seek employment, is not necessarily a neurotic choice. The absence of adequate alternatives such as private medical insurance or a national health care plan, often makes this the only apparent solution. This dilemma creates psychological and social problems which are difficult to treat and it imposes an obligation upon society to seek better resolution of the problem.

While they are of graver potential consequences, the problems of drug experimentation, habituation, and addiction apparently occur at no greater frequency than in the general population; however, data to substantiate this impression are not available. The problem of drug overuse is difficult to assess and to manage for several reasons: (1) pain is a recurring or chronic symptom of this disease, hence pain relief is a basic tenet of treatment; (2) analgesics are introduced and used beneficially early in the child's life, creating some feeling of dependency upon them; (3) individuals vary widely in their pain thresholds which are difficult to assess objectively, thus, the pain from past hemorrhagic episodes may be inadequately relieved leading to pain inducing anxiety with each new episode; or (4) the patient may have received insufficient early preparation for the reality that he must learn to tolerate some pain without depending upon drugs. Many of the drug problems of the late teen or young adult group are not unique to hemophilia but reflect the current "drug culture" aspects of society. Early counseling, on-going psychotherapy, psychiatric consultation as needed, and alternate facilities for detoxification and follow-up care are essential to manage satisfactorily the severe manifestations of this problem.

An individual's arrest for misdemeanor or felony charges may prompt him to attempt to use his hemophilic condition to avoid penalty or to receive preferential legal disposition. The Center staff provides information about hemophilia and its management to law enforcement officials and encourages equitable judicial disposition without regard for the hemophilia.

PREVENTIVE MENTAL HYGIENE

The need for psychological treatment of problems associated with hemophilia can be reduced considerably if parents and professional personnel adopt attitudes and measures to aid the boy toward a positive acceptance of his disease and of himself. Very early in the child's life, these factors must be considered:

(1) The basic needs for the satisfactory emotional development of the boy with hemophilia are the same as those of any other boy; first, he is an individual and second, he has hemophilia.

(2) His growth toward independence and satisfactory masculine identification requires the active participation of both his father and his mother or adequate parent substitutes.

(3) Parents must recognize that no matter how rigid their supervision of him, the boy will have hemorrhages as the result of engaging in those day to day activities which are necessary for his normal physical and emotional development.

(4) If the boy is given sufficient opportunity in the preschool years to discover those activities in which he can engage safely, he will soon discover for himself the cause and effect relationships between some activities and hemorrhages; thus, he will develop a sense of responsibility and independence and an acceptance of his limitations.

(5) Parents and medical staff should encourage his active participation in the evaluation of a hemorrhage or related condition.

(6) The boy will develop a sense of confidence and power when he recognizes that he can control the consequences of his hemophilia by selecting appropriate activities, by obtaining prompt treatment when hemorrhages occur, and by keeping himself in good physical condition through exercise. At a young age, he can learn that it is his knee, ankle, or elbow hemorrhage and that he has the right and the responsibility to participate in decisions about its management.

(7) Beginning in early childhood, he will be better able to manage his disease knowledgeably if he is given maximum information about hemophilia and he will feel more secure in educating others when the situation demands.

(8) Hopefully, the boy with hemophilia will recognize that he is essentially like other boys except for his deficient clotting factor. He can participate in most peer activities with some occasional modification of a specific activity. He will require prophylactic plasma concentrate administration for special events and he will need strong musculature to reduce the crippling deformities residual to his disease.

PSYCHOLOGICAL AND SOCIAL IMPLICATIONS OF THE HOME TRANSFUSION PROGRAM

The home transfusion program greatly relieves the family unit, especially the boy and his parents, from many of the identified stresses. Family activities, school, and other important events are not disrupted by frequent, untimely trips to the Center for outpatient plasma therapy or for hospital admission. Since plasma therapy can be fitted more conveniently into the family routine, life becomes more predictable for the patient and his family. They experience a reduction of recriminations, anxiety, pressures, and guilt. When securing treatment for himself no longer causes great family inconvenience, the child feels freer to indicate the occurrence of a hemorrhage and to treat it himself or assist with the infusion. Both he and his parents develop greater feelings of independence, confidence, and responsibility in managing hemorrhagic episodes whether at home or away. Siblings, who remained at home or were excluded from hospital treatment areas, become familiar with and accepting of the treatment procedures. By the time the boy has reached his middle teen years, he will be secure and confident about leaving home to attend college or to accept employment since he can proficiently assess and treat most of his usual hemorrhages.

GENETIC COUNSELING

Professional efforts with patients and family members in genetic counseling may be doomed to failure or may encounter massive resistance, if they do not take into account the individual's *basic right* to decide for himself about procreation, marriage, abortion, and adoption. While factual genetic information should be given repeatedly by all staff members at appropriate times, the individual's feelings, wishes and personal needs must be recognized and respected. The carrier daughter or sister of the hemophiliac should be appraised of her carrier status as completely as possible. When and how this information is given will vary with the situation, but it should be shared with an awareness of the girl's emotional maturity and receptiveness as well as with a sensitivity to her reactions to the information. These same considerations are important in counseling the young male adult. He should know that *all* of his daughters will be obligatory carriers. If he feels personally unfulfilled with few successful or gratifying experiences, conceiving and parenting a child may be of tremendous importance to him. If his or the carrier's decision, resulting in a new generation of carriers or hemophiliacs, was made in spite of strong advice and warnings by the genetic counselor, the latter has failed in his intended purpose and may have contributed measurably to guilt feelings

and other stresses in the new generation. If, on the other hand, the individual was given complete information and was treated with dignity and respect, he or she will have worked toward a decision appropriate for him or her and will be more amenable to further consultation.

SUMMARY

The occurrence of hemophilia in a family imposes stresses upon the family unit and upon each of its members. Unless these social and psychological stresses associated with the disease are understood and treated early in his development, the individual with hemophilia may suffer severe emotional handicaps in adulthood. Disabling problems of excessive dependency, emotional immaturity, low self-esteem, impulsive and self-destructive behavior, and so forth all have their beginnings in early childhood, a period in which many important personality features are formed. The adult's most important and long lasting feelings about himself come from his parents' earlier attitudes and feelings toward him and toward one another, and from their relationship with him during his formative years. If their feelings and actions are characterized by acceptance, affection, support, and assurance, he will become more able to deal effectively with the unique stresses and limitations imposed upon him by hemophilia.

The comprehensive management of hemophilia demands timely and adequate medical care to minimize the occurrence of physical disability. Likewise, it requires prophylactic mental hygiene counseling, psychological evaluation and psychotherapy as needed, and educational and vocational counseling to minimize the occurrence of psychosocial disabilities. Ideally, the professional personnel providing these services should function as members of a multidiscipline team, through a Center which provides basic care for hemophilia. In this setting, they can become more aware of all aspects of the disease, can acquire a longitudinal understanding of each patient and his family, and can be more readily available to other personnel for consultation.

The psychotherapeutic methods utilized for treating individuals with hemophilia and members of their families are not unique, although the psychotherapist should have an appreciation of the unique stresses of hemophilia upon various family members. Family therapy and brief-term therapy are frequently used approaches, with periodic follow-up evaluations during childhood and adolescence. Brief-term supportive counseling for the individual and his family members may be of crucial importance at various stages of his life, such as entry into school, adolescence, adulthood, marriage, and employment. With early brief-term treatment and follow-up, a great majority of individuals function within normal limits, despite the many complications imposed by the disease. A small percentage require long-term psychotherapy and a still smaller percentage may require intensive inpatient psychiatric care, some of the latter because of drug dependency or addiction.

Because the home transfusion program greatly relieves many of the stresses experienced by the boy and his parents in securing timely and appropriate treatment, its contributions to improved mental hygiene in the family are readily apparent. Furthermore, because the boy has learned at an early age that he can successfully assess and treat hemorrhagic episodes, he is able to enter adulthood with greater confidence and security.

REFERENCES

1. Agle, D. P.: Psychiatric Complications of Hemophilia, in Brinkhous, Kenneth (ed.): *The Hemophilias*. University of North Carolina Press, Chapel Hill, 1964.
2. Bittner, E: *Your Child and Hemophilia*. Los Angeles Orthopaedic Hospital, Los Angeles, 1974.
3. Katz, A. H.: *Hemophilia: A Study in Hope and Reality*. Charles C Thomas, Springfield, 1970.

12

REHABILITATION COUNSELING

Charlotte Taylor

Mr. H., age 58, has severe hemophilia A with marked degenerative changes in his spine and in all major joints. In an interview, Mr. H. talks about his 30 years of work as an architectural draftsman. "I like my work. My boss likes it too. He won't let anyone else touch the drawings for the new contract. A couple of weeks ago I had so much pain—I had been awake all night—I called in to say that I couldn't make it in to work and the boss said, 'Can you come down at all and just sit at the desk and handle phone calls?' After I went down, I didn't feel the pain as much, and that's the truth."

The majority of men with hemophilia have work that is safe and reasonably satisfying. Some, like Mr. H., have work that they savor. But approximately one out of four working age hemophiliacs in this country is not working or is in a highly unsatisfactory work situation.[1,2] In this chapter, material from case histories and taped interviews is used to illustrate problems that interfere with healthy vocational development and adjustment. The counseling skills and techniques that are described in the management of these problems are particularly appropriate when counseling with patients in a hospital setting where supportive services from a hemophilia treatment team are available.

At the Regional Hemophilia Center the rehabilitation counselor's case load comprises adolescent and adult clients who need help with school adjustment, career choice, job training, job placement, and retirement. The counseling relationship in the Center continues over a longer period of time than it would in an agency or in an acute care setting, for example, hemophilic boys at the Center have been counseled from junior high school into college or job entry, and adults, from working status into retirement. This sustained counseling relationship has the potential to modify the patient role which usually is characterized by passivity, an acceptance of authority, and a willingness to surrender autonomy. The sustained relationship also provides an opportunity for the counselor to use a wide variety of skills, techniques, and services and to examine their effectiveness through longitudinal study.

SKILLS, TECHNIQUES, AND SERVICES

Interviewing

A skill that stands out as an important determinant in the success of the vocational rehabilitation process is the counselor's ability to assess how circumstances in the client's life affect his vocational decisions. This skill develops as the counselor learns to communicate with the client in ways that illuminate the details and meaning of these circumstances. One effective technique is to allow the client to guide the course of the interview. By using what the client says to maintain continuity, the counselor learns what the client chooses to talk about and how he chooses to present himself. Consider the clues to his identification model, to the imprints and demands of his parents, and to his life style in meeting problems in these excerpts from an interview with 17-year-old Miguel who aspires to be a jazz musician (electric bass). Miguel responds to the question, "What's it like in your family?" with:

"I've got a father and a mother, you know, the standard equipment. My father does the usual father things. He works. He was a big-band musician back in the '50s, so naturally he thinks I'm just following the most perfect course in the universe in being a musician. That's good, too. I like that. He doesn't bother me about anything. It goes back to when he wore zoot suits when *he* was age 17. My hair's just the same thing. It doesn't phase him at all. He knows that there are some nights when I will come back from a night's practice with my group at 2 a.m., dead tired, and he's not going to hassle me because I came in at 2 o'clock. . . . My mother, on the other hand is the exact opposite, which upsets me. I think most hemophiliac's mothers have such a complex of protecting their little boys, they won't accept that they grow up. You know, they just can't accept that. Like, I came home and said that I was checking into applying to _____ College. I said, 'If I go, I'm going to have to live there.' You should have seen the bawling fit she had! She was bawling all over the house. I haven't even applied yet and she was ready to jump over the Grand Canyon. I can't have that. The split's going to be awful. . . ."

In a second excerpt from the interview, Miguel talks about his feelings concerning his right foot, which has been deformed by recurring pseudotumors. (See case history in Chapter 8, p. 95.)

"My hands are great, but this foot isn't functional and it bleeds all the time. I can't stand on it. If I do, the muscle gives out. I tell them (the doctors) 'Hey, why don't you do your thing (amputate the foot) and I can get on with my plans.' But naturally, they say, 'No, because we're going to recon-

struct your foot in five years.' Five years!!!"

Counselors may find it frustrating to have to consider the many factors in the complex interrelationship between the biophysical, social, and psychological forces in the client's life before making a vocational diagnosis or developing a plan for services. This is particularly the case when the need for employment is pressing. However, short cuts usually result in a recycling of the client through vocational rehabilitation services.

Testing

Test data can be a valuable adjunct to life history data in evaluation areas that are of critical importance in guidance, that is, intelligence, interests, aptitudes, performance, and personality dynamics. A diagnostic picture, to be of great help in counseling, should be accompanied by therapeutic skill in interpretation and by an administrative climate that appreciates the values of intensive counseling. At this Center, educational and vocational diagnostic tests are administered on an "as needed" basis. Those used most frequently are: the Wechsler Adult Intelligence Scale, the Wechsler Intelligence Scale for Children, the Differential Aptitude Tests, the General Aptitudes Tests Battery, the Kuder Vocational Preference Record, the Strong Interests Blank, the Wide Range Achievement Test, the Minnesota Multiphasic Personality Inventory, the Forer Sentence Completion Test, and the Guilford Zimmerman Temperament Survey.

In 1968, testing data used for counseling purposes at the Center were compiled to establish norms for intelligence quotients, for achievement levels, and for profiles of interest and personality.[2] These results are described below.

Intelligence

Seventy-eight clients, ages 16 to 50, were given the Wechsler Adult Intelligence Scale. The full scale mean score

Table 12-1. Intelligence quotients (n=78)

	Verbal	Performance	Full scale
Mean	116.6	115.3	116.7
Range of I.Q.s	70–140	85–137	75–140

Table 12-2. Wide range achievement quotients (n=78)

	Reading	Spelling	Arithmetic
Mean	111.46	95.33	93.29
Range of WRAT	70–158	62–141	71–149

for this group is 116.7 (bright-normal range of intelligence). This mean is significantly higher than that of normal population ($P < 0.001$). Intelligence quotients are shown in Table 12-1.

Achievement

Seventy-eight clients, ages 7 to 20, were given the Wide Range Achievement Test (WRAT). These quotients are shown in Table 12-2.

Based on a normal population average of 100, the group placed at the 78th percentile in reading, the 38th percentile in spelling, and the 46th percentile in arithmetic. Their levels of achievement in spelling and arithmetic were significantly lower than would be expected in terms of their I.Q.s. These results are consistent with those obtained by Olch[3] in 1971 in her study of the "Effects of Hemophilia Upon Intellectual Growth and Academic Achievement." Although Olch's study did not confirm a relationship between low achievement and poor school attendance, we feel that school absences do play a large part in the achievement deficiencies of the patient group served at the Center. Reading skills do not suffer proportionately because they are used more frequently in out of school situations and tend to be maintained at a level closest to capacity. These skills are also more closely related to intelligence. Students participating in the Home Tranfusion Program have markedly improved their school attendance. A longitudinal study that began at the time of their initial testing for intelligence and achievement will further clarify the relationship between school attendance and achievement level.

Interests

The Strong Vocational Interest Blank was used to measure the client's interests in a manner that allowed him to compare his likes and dislikes with those of individuals in specified occupations. Results in five occupational areas are shown in Table 12-3. Career interests most frequently expressed by hemophilic clients served at the Center are in medicine, social work, and psychology. (Nearly all disabled groups of people show significantly high social service interests.) It seems reasonable that hemophiliacs would identify with the professional people who have helped them. Moreover, they might hope to find relief from their own physical and psychological pain in the human services role. While we would agree with Katz[1] that human services occupations offer attractive and suitable careers to hemophiliacs, the counselor should try to learn whether the choice is realistic or unhealthy and whether it will lead to vocational adjustment or will amplify emotional stress.

Two nonoccupational scores on the Strong Vocational Interest Blank were analyzed: Occupational Level and Masculinity-Feminity. The high score on the Occupational Level scale indicates that the client's responses were similar to those of most professionals and businessmen. The mean of the standard scores for the Masculinity-Femininity Index indicates typically masculine inter-

Table 12-3. Strong vocational interest blanks

	C					C+	B−	B	B+	A		
	0	5	10	15	20	25	30	35	40	45	50	55	60
Biological science													
Engineering and physical science						├──	──	┼──	──	┤			
Social services					├──	──	┼──	──	┤				
Business				├──	──	┼──	──	┤					
Sales				├──	──	──	┼──	──	┤				
Occupational level					├──	──	┼──	──	┤				
Masculinity-femininity									├──	┼──	┤		

A rating = interest similar to that of people successfully engaged in these areas.

est. In this regard, the findings from a study by Weise[4] have provocative implications for vocational counseling; hemophiliacs appeared to perceive as feminine those occupations which limit physical activity. They opt for occupations involving a high level of physical activity because they perceive these as masculine.

The findings from our studies of intelligence and of interests patterns have been substantiated by investigators working elsewhere with hemophiliacs[3,6] but general inferences must await further research.

Personality

The Minnesota Multiphasic Personality Inventory was administered to 64 clients aged 14 to 57; 53 of these were adolescents and young adults under the age of 25 years. Of the clients 32 were hospitalized at the time of testing. Hospitalized and outpatients were evenly distributed over the two age groups. No significant differences were found when the mean scores of the scales of hospitalized and nonhospitalized clients were compared.

Neither the adolescent nor the adult group showed any major disturbance. The profile for the juveniles suggested that they were discharging anger and rebellion against the restraints and frustrations imposed on them by hemophilia by freely acting out. (There was little to suggest that this noncompliant behavior was counterphobic.) The adults were higher on the depression scale than the adolescents and appeared to internalize anxiety and stress by coping through intellectualization and repression. Both adolescents and adults revealed a deficiency in the ability to socialize and to handle interpersonal relationships. However, the defensive structure was intact and ego functioning was not threatened. Agle's findings[5] were similar; psychological disorder seen in hemophiliacs can be as varied as there are psychological entities but rarely is there psychosis.

The chief value of the normative data, described above, is their contribution towards a better understanding of the clients served at this Center, that is, a clearer picture of the disparity between the adolescent's good intelligence and his poor academic achievement has provided insights into his acting out behavior and has led to services that direct the boy's energy towards attainable goals.

Team Practice

Kahn,[7] speaking of team practice, says that team members are expected to share appropriate information about the patient's situation with mutual benefit and to share in the direction of the treatment program. She points out that effective collaboration also requires that team members share with each other new knowledge from education and research in their field. This builds the knowledge base of each team member in the area of interrelationships between the biophysical, social, and psychological factors.

There are obstacles to this kind of communication. Each team member has a need for recognition that affects his willingness to share the responsibility for the client's care with his coworkers. These domain conflicts are sometimes expressed by withholding information from fellow workers about the client's situation or from the client about the availability of other services on the team. Domain conflicts are less frequent when team members continually raise the level of knowledge and practice skills in their specialty. This tends to clarify roles and functions and makes each worker feel more secure about releasing generic tasks to other members of the team.

The problem-oriented medical record (POMR) can serve as a basic mechanism for keeping each team member aware of the others' treatment plans and insights, and of the patient's progress. The POMR is a patient-oriented system of charting whereby entries focus on problems and efforts to solve them. The system has four components: data base (physical and psychosocial factors), problem list (supported by the data base), plans for treatment or management, and progress notes. Problems are numbered and titled; new information is numbered and titled to match the problems to which it relates. The POMR encourages accountability for good judgement and performance of team members.

Specialized evaluations of the client by other disciplines on the team are essential aids to the counselor for vocational assessment and problem solving, that is, the occupational therapist is a resource for perceptual motor testing for the diagnosis of learning problems, and for prevocational testing to assess gross and fine dexterity, work habits, eye-hand coordination, clerical skills, and tool handling. The physical therapist provides the counselor with information about the client's range of joint motion, muscle strength, and functional abilities, and recommends devices to assist in the performance of specific tasks. The psychiatric social worker shares insights about the client's intrapsychic and family strengths (or problems) that need to be considered in vocational planning. Throughout the vocational rehabilitation process, the physicians on the team define and monitor the client's medical care program and serve as consultants to the counselor regarding the client's physical status and prognosis. Team member involvement and cooperation in vocational rehabilitation are demonstrated in the following letters. The first letter, prepared by a physician on the Center team, illustrates the use of medical information to educate an employer about a potential hemophilic employee.

Mr. _____
Personnel Director
_____ Telephone Company
_____ , California

Mr. _____ is applying for a position with _____ Telephone Company. As you know, Mr. _____ has hemophilia. Hemophilia is such a rare and unique condition that he thought it would be helpful for you to know what it is and what it is not, so that you could better evaluate his physical qualifications for the job.

The person with hemophilia has little or none of a plasma protein needed to form a clot. For this reason, it takes a long time for a clot to form. When the clot does form, it is soft and mushy and isn't an effective plug for the blood vessel. For this reason, people with hemophilia have prolonged bleeding from deep cuts, large bruises, and bleeding into joints. They do *not* bleed any faster than normal people. This bleeding can be prevented or controlled by giving the missing clotting factor in the form of plasma concentrate. Mr. _____ can administer his own concentrate, very much as a diabetic would administer insulin.

Last April, Mr. _____ had hip surgery to correct an orthopedic disability caused by bleeding into the hip joint. Limitations of motion as a result of this surgery should not interfere with office work of any kind.

Mr. _____ is known to the Hemophilia Center team as a responsible, resourceful, and bright young man. We feel that he is an excellent candidate for job training for your company.

If we can be of further help in answering any questions that you have about Mr. _____ or about hemophilia, please let us know.

The second letter was written by the psychiatric social worker in response to a rehabilitation counselor's concern about his client's psychosexual development.

Mr. _____
Rehabilitation Counselor
State Department of Rehabilitation
_____, California

I am writing to provide a summary of my evaluation of Mr. Allen D. As a psychiatric social worker on the Hemophilia Rehabilitation Center staff, I have known Allen for the past four years. I saw him for an 8 month period of supportive psychotherapy in addition to intermittent interviews when he has come to Orthopaedic Hospital for inpatient or outpatient care. I would like to review some details of his personal and family history so that you may better understand his current adjustment and the progress that he has made in recent years.

Allen, age 29, lives with his father, age 78, and his mother, 65. His father is a quiet man who worked long hours on his date ranch before retirement. He was content to let his wife take a dominant role in family life and felt relieved

that she could manage the difficult problems presented by their son's hemophilia. He regarded Allen as more or less an "invalid," unable to help him with ranch chores, and in recent years as an inadequate adult, essentially dependent on family. . . .

Early in psychotherapy, Allen's feeling of low self-esteem, his passivity, excessive caution, self-doubt, and delayed psychosexual development were very much in evidence. He was also extremely inhibited verbally, evidencing little of his superior intelligence (WAIS index 130). He passively resisted many attempts to become more independent, but gradually gained insight into his wish to remain dependent. . . . As psychotherapy progressed and with a maximum of emotional support from other rehabilitation team members during a long hospitalization, Allen began to assume confidence. He participated actively in his physical therapy program and was able to relate meaningfully and comfortably with people outside of his own family. He showed an appropriate and healthy interest in members of the opposite sex, which was sometimes "adolescent" in manifestation but nonetheless indicated that his self-concept was changing and that he regarded himself as masculine. Allen continues in this positive direction through his interest in pictures in Playboy magazine. I believe that you mentioned that someone had referred to this interest as "pornographic." On the contrary, I believe that this represents a healthy and developing part of this man's personality.

Allen has taken an increasingly active and responsible role in moving toward realistic vocational plans. I feel tremendously pleased about your interest in helping him to develop these. . . . He needs your encouragement and support and he also needs continued help from us. I am very glad to have the opportunity to work closely together with you in this. . . .

In letters such as these, the experiences

and insights of the Center staff have provided health care professionals in the community with new frames of reference for working with hemophilic patients.

The counselor who works on a hemophilia team inevitably witnesses trauma, suffering, and death. These create conscious or unconscious feelings of inadequacy, guilt, identification, and grief. These feelings are difficult to manage, particularly by oneself. One of the most important ways that team members serve one another is through the sharing of feelings as a mutual support system.

Work Evaluation

The assessment of employability factors through the use of work, real or simulated, is a useful technique when other standard assessment techniques have failed to generate a plan of action. Work evaluation focuses on general employability factors such as social development, work habits, physical tolerance, performance rate, and on specific employability factors such as skills, aptitudes, dexterities, and intelligence. Methods of work evaluation commonly available on a referral basis in the community are work samples, sheltered workshops, and actual work conditions. Work sampling is usually carried out in the work evaluation units of rehabilitation facilities. The work samples may be actual jobs administered and observed under standard conditions, or mock-ups of a component of a job. Work sample evaluation has some special advantages: it is less influenced than psychological tests by language inadequacies, reading disabilities, educational deprivation, or cultural differences. Sampling is an especially useful method for determining safe limits for those hemophilic clients who are interested in jobs that require strenuous physical activity or the use of heavy equipment or tools.

Sheltered workshops simulate actual working conditions. These conditions, regular working hours, wages, etc., more closely resemble those of industry and business than do work samples. Evaluations at sheltered workshops are limited by the workshop's contracts, usually involving products consisting of simple assembly tasks. In general, sheltered workshops have not been appropriate for assessing the skills and work potential of clients served at this Center. Many otherwise well motivated clients have found the general setting of the workshop a threat to their self-esteem. Except for the mentally retarded and marginal worker, the wages paid to workshop clients are not a realistic incentive for the average hemophiliac, who is brighter and more dextrous than the average industrial worker. (Fine precision skills reflect the high experience level of hemophiliacs in hobbies that require precise hand use.[8]) In the following case the client was an appropriate candidate for referral and has benefited from his workshop experience.

Harry P., age 31, has severe hemophilia A and severe left hemiplegia and organic brain damage from cerebral vascular accidents at age 2 and age 15. He did not attend school and had only sporadic bedside teaching during his numerous hospitalizations. Mr. P. tests in the dull-normal range of intelligence but at the time of his referral to a sheltered workshop, he could neither read nor write. He was wheelchair bound, lived in a custodial home and had never been employed. As a hobby he assembled model cars, a feat he performed with considerable skill despite his virtually useless left hand. He enjoyed watching cooking lessons on T.V. and wished that he had an opportunity to prepare his own meals. He expressed a strong desire to break away from supervised care and to live independently.

In order to use public transportation to the workshop, he needed to be able to walk. Special shoes were prescribed by the team's orthopedist; his walking training was conducted by the physical therapist. Initially a mock-up of bus steps was used for practice in getting on and off the bus. Later he was accompanied by the physical therapist on "dry-run" trips to the workshop until he was able to recognize the appropriate buses and to manage bus transfers alone.

Progress reports from the workshop indicated good ability to function under supervised instruction and improvement in social skills, but poor attention to the task at hand. The problem? Mr. P. was in love with the girl who sat across from him at the work table. His work rate did not improve. After a year he was dismissed from the workshop as "unmotivated."

He was referred to another workshop and made good progress initially. Again he became infatuated with a coworker and was dismissed.

There were many gains during these workshop experiences: Mr. P. had moved into an apartment, and was managing his own personal care and business affairs. He had taken a workshop sponsored class in remedial reading and arithmetic and could read at the third grade level. (His primer was the California Motor Vehicle Code.) He banked enough money to buy a car, and, coached by the Center's rehabilitation counselor, passed the written examination and the driver's test.

Presently Mr. P. has requested help in finding new workshop placement; he wants to earn money to buy car insurance. Before referring him to another workshop, the counselor will focus on helping Mr. P. to express and gratify his affectional needs in more appropriate ways. Another "crush" at work will defeat his goal to earn money to maintain his car.

Occupational Information

A lack of knowledge of work opportunities adds to the hemophilic client's employment handicap. Occupational information can broaden the range of his job choice, help him to locate the chosen occupation, and guide his training. It can also sharpen the possibilities that his needs will be satisfied and that his aptitudes will find expression within the context of a particular job.

The counselor's sources of occupational information are his own stock of information acquired from counseling and placement activities and from personal contacts with key people in industry and in trade schools. Formal references, such as the Dictionary of Occupational Titles (D.O.T.),[9] Occupational Outlook Handbook,[10] job monographs, bulletins, special releases, and documentary films should be part of his library.

An immediate, practical source of occupational information can be obtained by subscribing to occupational guides which are regularly revised in the light of current trends. In California, an excellent publication of this sort is The Occupational Guide. Leaflets, pamphlets and monographs published by the Department of Labor are usually accurate and free from bias.

In our experience, the D.O.T. is an indispensable reference for use in comparing the client's profile with that of the job. It can be an especially valuable aid in uncovering clues for job possibilities that the client will also see as possibilities if the counselor is knowledgeable about the more subtle aspects of jobs and about how these fit with the "inner world" of the client. If, for example, the job involves pressure, does the client go to pieces under a deadline, or is he the kind of person who creates a deadline just to start the adrenalin pouring?

In using occupational information with clients at the Center, the counselor has found these guidelines to be important. (1) The client should be informed of trends in the labor market and of the employment outlook for jobs that he is considering. (2) The counselor should be careful about unconscious expression of bias; material should be objectively and dispassionately presented and the client given an opportunity to express his feelings about it. (3) The counselor should not insist that the client's career goals be "realistic." Present striving can be worthwhile, even though it is aimed at future goals that seem to be set unrealistically high. (4) The counselor should not teach the client about occupations, but involve him in learning about them. An especially valuable way to do this is to provide the client with an opportunity to observe people at work in occupations that interest him. This is illustrated by the following case excerpt:

Doug L. has hemophilia B. He functions quite well physically despite motion restrictions in his knees and elbows. He is an outgoing, friendly, witty 17 year old, gifted in verbal and written communication skills. At school he has won recognition for writing satire and drawing cartoons for the school paper and magazine.

During vocational counseling, Doug expressed a keen interest in advertising as a career, a choice that was strongly supported by counseling and testing. In a counseling session with Doug and his father, his father commented that he thought that advertising was just one more of Doug's "crazy ideas" about what he wanted to do. (Previous "crazy ideas" included journalism, law, T.V. sales, and psychology professor.)

Arrangements were made for Doug to spend a day with an advertising agency executive who introduced him to agency personnel at work and demonstrated the ways in which advertising relates to marketing, public relations, and sales promotions.

Following this day in the field, the counselor found Doug exuberant over the discovery that advertising included so many activities that he liked. This provided an opportunity to review the "crazy ideas" list and to point out that it was made up of occupations that are similar in aptitudes and interests to many jobs in the advertising field. Doug was pleased and his father relieved by this interpretation.

Client Advocacy

Any team member may serve as the patient's/client's advocate in order to help him to get all available services from community resources. The counselor frequently assumes the advocacy role in making contacts with school, agency, and employment personnel on behalf of the client. These contacts also serve to help the community develop an awareness of the "hemophilia experience" and to change stereotypes and attitudes.

School

One of the responsibilities of the rehabilitation counselor is to take an active part in working with school personnel to establish a stable school setting and a program suitable to the developmental and academic needs of the individual student. Attendance at a regular public school is encouraged. Referrals are made for home, tele-teaching, or hospital teaching programs during those periods when the student is incapacitated. We have found that regular public schools or schools that integrate handicapped and nonhandicapped students are safe for the hemophilic student and that they offer a richer curriculum and a greater opportunity for positive school experience than do schools for the handicapped. We are guided by the principle that hemophilic children should be placed where they can be best educated at the least distance from the mainstream of society. If they must be sent to a restricted school, programs should be aimed at eventually integrating them into a public school. In 1970, only 17 children in our school aged patient group of 220 patients were attending schools for the handicapped in contrast to 33 children in a school aged patient group of 140 patients in 1964.

Necessary changes are handled most effectively when the rehabilitation counselor and other members of the hemophilia team meet in person with school personnel. Ideally, everyone responsible for the boy's care, including the boy himself, should participate in the conference: the school physician, principal, teacher, nurse, guidance counselor, and their professional counterparts on the Center team. The role of the rehabilitation counselor in these conferences is to make recommendations for developmental and remedial academic programs and for classroom or campus adaptations that will permit the use of assistive devices, e.g., crutches, wheelchair, or splints. Specific suggestions frequently made are that: (1) the boy be given a duplicate set of books so that he need not carry them to and from school and so that one set is always at home in case of absence, (2) repetitive stair climbing be reduced by scheduling as many classes as possible on one level, (3) physical education classes be adapted to the boy's exercise program (rather than have him spend this time in study hall or in other sedentary activity) and, (4) he be allowed to take classes in wood-shop, biology, chemistry, etc., since possible nicks and cuts from handling equipment do not constitute a danger and can be treated by applying normal first aid measures.

Experience with the Home Transfusion Program at this Center and recent studies[11,12,13] indicate a dramatic decrease in school absences when hemorrhages are managed by home treatment programs. If absences continue when quality treatment is available, the therapy may be inadequate, the boy or his family may not be making optimal use of the program, or the boy may be using his hemophilia to avoid school.

Work Experience

Almost any kind of work experience can be valuable for the hemophilic teenager. If for wages so much the better, but participation in Junior Achievement and Work Experience programs in the community and in library and office work at school are possibilities that the rehabilitation counselor and the school counselor can help the boy to explore.

At the Center, the counselor has developed resources in private industry for part-time work and job training in such areas as data processing, film processing, orthodontia appliance assembly and repair, merchandise display, valet parking, theater ushering, grocery boxing, typing and filing, short-order cooking, and installing automobile accessories.

Successful part-time work experience depends heavily on family and Center-team support; the boy will need cooperation and endorsement of his plans, that is, assurance that he will get plasma or other care to manage bleeding episodes that may result from increased activity and a treatment regimen that is scheduled around his work hours.

Training

Research shows that people who are most at ease with the society today, most pleased with their work, gratified with their income, and content with their personal lives are those who are working in professional, managerial, and technical positions. This dramatizes the plight of hemophiliacs who are working in low level blue collar jobs or who are not working at all. In talking with them, one realizes that the idea of meaningful work is as attractive as to the college educated, but they do not really expect to find it without specialized training or a college education. Counseling the hemophilic client to examine the opportunities for self-fulfillment, financial reward, and autonomy in the kind of work that is open to him with further training, carries with it the responsibility of helping him to find viable ways to solve practical, reality problems that may stand in the way of the decision to continue training. Problems of this nature that are frequently confronted in counseling are the client's need for a high school diploma as a prerequisite to further training; training resources and subsidies for maintenance and medical care during the training period; equal opportunity in hiring practices (All that education, for what?); finances to cover the cost of medical care once he is employed and no longer eligible for state medical aid.

If the client is 18 years old or older and is a high school dropout, he may earn a high school equivalency certificate or 80 elective credits towards a high school diploma by taking the General Educational Development test. He may prepare for this test through programmed instruction in labs or small study groups in community adult education centers. The instruction is usually available in day or evening classes on an open enrollment basis that allows flexibility in scheduling classes to fit in with full or part-time work.

Persons with hemophilia who are unemployed are usually eligible for vocational rehabilitation services sponsored by the state. In California this agency is the Department of Rehabilitation. In some states, the vocational rehabilitation agency is associated with the state education agency; in others it is organized as a separate commission or department. Office of Vocational Rehabilitation, Bureau of Vocational Rehabilitation, or Division of Vocational Rehabilitation are names by which these agencies are known.

Services available through the many local offices of the agency are: evaluation, counseling, medical and therapeutic care, prosthetic and orthotic devices, training, maintenance and transportation, tools, equipment and licenses, and placement. When clients served by this Center are referred to the Department of Rehabilitation, the Center counselor assists in evaluating their vocational needs and abilities. The client who has directed himself toward a career choice before applying to the agency usually moves quickly into a job training or college program sponsored by the agency. In some states, the client may receive Supplementary Security Income (SSI) while he is in a training program if he is financially eligible. Income from part-time work is not deducted from SSI benefits during the training period, provided that it can be shown that such income is necessary for self-support while the client is in training.

Job Placement

Job placement of the hemophilic client is the capstone of the evaluation procedures and of the case services that have prepared him for employment. The majority of clients who have received vocational rehabilitation services at the Center have taken the initiative in locating job possibilities. Talking persuasively and honestly about one's experience, skills, and interests to the person who has the power to hire is the most effective tool for finding work. Rehearsing the interview by role playing in counseling sessions can be helpful preparation.

In some instances, clients have requested the counselor to "interpret" hemophilia to prospective employers, company physicians, or insurance carriers; in others, they have handled the interpretation very well alone. In either case, the message is given that improved medical procedures, chiefly patient administered concentrates, and prescribed exercise have greatly improved the probability that hemophiliacs can carry out safely the physical demands of their jobs and keep work absences at an acceptable level.

There is, of course, no list of jobs suitable for the hemophilic worker, but if he is to be safe from work injuries and able to maintain good work attendance, he will need a supporting environment that ideally includes these factors: (1) employer's knowledge of the worker's hemophilia and accurate and current information about the disorder, (2) coverage by the company's group medical insurance, (3) accessibility to the worker's treatment facilities, particularly if he is not on a self-infusion program, (4) avoidance of heavy lifting or the operation of heavy equipment, (5) permission to move about frequently to avoid stiffness and to use assistive devices whenever necessary, (6) access to elevators and ramps when necessary. Clients at the Center frequently express a double bind conflict about concealing their hemophilia from employers: if they disclose their condition, they chance being refused jobs because hemophiliacs are considered high injury risks; if they conceal their hemophilia, they encounter serious problems. For example, they are (1) unable to get plasma therapy or medical care during working hours, (2) unable to avail themselves of company sponsored health insurance plans for treatment of hemophilia, (3) assigned unwittingly to hazardous jobs, and (4) put under an emotional strain by the subterfuge. This strain not only adversely affects relations with employers and colleagues but it may also be precursive to work accidents.

An extreme example of the effect that concealment can have on the outcome of a work injury is illustrated in the following experience of a client served by the Center:

Mr. C., 30, has mild classic hemophilia. He is a robust, muscular man who until his injury had a continuous work history in manual labor jobs. Three and a half years ago, while working as a rubbish collector, a paper bag containing a cement block and part of an iron post burst open with the block hitting his knee. His knee became swollen and painful. He reported the injury to the company's physician but did not reveal that he had hemophilia lest it come to the attention of his employer. Mr. C.'s leg was placed in a cast. Six weeks later there were severe medical complications necessitating surgery. At this time he felt constrained to reveal his hemophilia.

Mr. C. had two surgical procedures requiring long hospitalizations. Medical and other benefits have been paid by

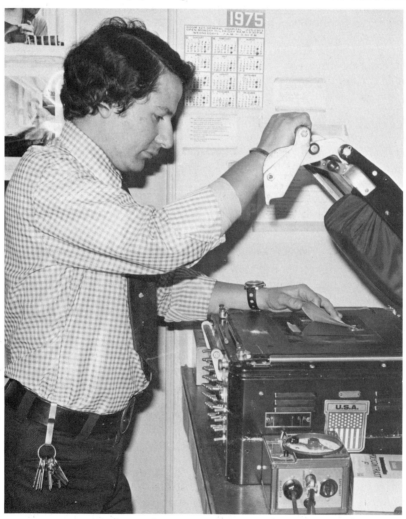

Figure 12-1. Patient at work: Most of his printing involves use of the contact printer. Micrographs, X-rays, graphs, charts, and identification pictures are prepared in this manner.

Workmen's Compensation insurance and by public welfare programs. These have been in excess of $20,000. Mr. C. is now physically able to train for work more suitable to his disability, but his lawyer has discouraged him from doing this, pending adjudication of the insurance claim.

In contrast to Mr. C.'s experience, there is the case of Robert, who has severe classic hemophilia:

Ten years ago when Robert requested rehabilitation counseling services at the Center, he was working sporadically as a freelance wedding and portrait photographer. He liked the work but was discouraged about continuing; invariably he bled on the day of an important assignment. Lifting and carrying heavy camera equipment exacerbated hemorrhaging into badly damaged shoulder, elbow, and knee joints.

Robert retrained in biologic and medical photography in on the job training programs at a medical center. He was hired by the medical center following the training period.

He uses photographic equipment in ways that increase his range of motion in

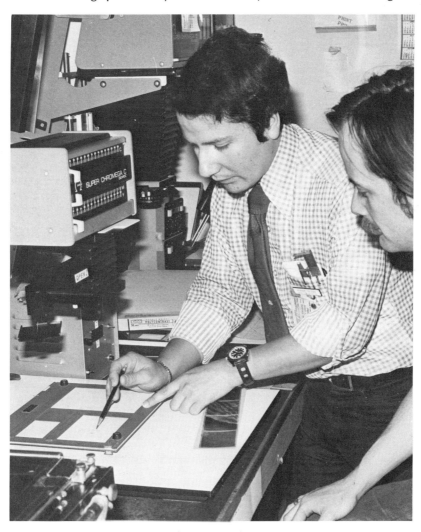

Figure 12-2. Patient at work: As darkroom supervisor, he works closely with his crew to answer their questions and to assure that each job is properly completed on time.

shoulders and arms (Fig. 12-1). He controls hemorrhages by self-administering concentrate from a supply that he keeps at work.

His work calls for continued growth in understanding and skills. It provides him with recognition, variety, and responsibility (Fig. 12-2).

A Study of Factors Associated with Work Injuries of Hemophiliacs in Southern California[14] found that workers with mild hemophilia are more apt to conceal their hemophilia and to work in blue collar jobs than are workers with severe hemophilia. White collar workers do not conceal their hemophilia as frequently because they are less likely to be rejected for employment on the basis of injury risk. (The relative hazards of a company's line of work are used for setting rates for Workmen's Compensation insurance; these rates are modified by the accident experience of the company.) Another reason why white collar workers do not conceal their hemophilia is that they cannot avoid disclosure of their condition; orthopedic impairments are too obvious and bleeding episodes too frequent. Hemophiliacs who wish to work in other than white collar jobs should not be forced to conceal their hemophilia, but neither should employers be expected to bear the full costs of compensating these workers for injury. A suggested solution to the problem is reform in Workmen's Compensation laws. For example, funds could be drawn from the State treasury to help defray the added costs of compensating a hemophiliac for injury. If legislation of this nature is passed, other measures such as Section 503 Rehabilitation Act of 1973 will be more effective in promoting the employment of hemophiliacs.

This act provides that every Federal agency contract of more than $2500 will include an affirmative action clause requiring that qualified handicapped applicants be actively recruited, considered, and employed. All qualified handicapped employees will be afforded nondiscriminatory consideration for promotion and job advancement. Individuals seeking the benefits of these programs need to make the fact of their handicap known to the employer to assure that the affirmative effort of an employer is directed to appropriate persons.

Disability Benefits

Hemophiliacs who are too severely disabled to engage in work activity may make application with the Social Security Administration for Social Security Disability Insurance (SSDI) or for Supplementary Security Income (SSI). SSDI and SSI are federal programs designed for the severely disabled who are unable to engage in competitive employment. SSDI is based on previous work history, whereas SSI is based solely on need factor. In both cases, persons can be helped through vocational rehabilitation counseling and/or retraining to prepare for and secure work which they can do.

Social Security Disability Insurance

To be eligible for SSDI the applicant must have paid into Social Security during his working years for a specified amount of time which is determined according to his age bracket. The benefit payments that he will receive from SSDI will be based essentially on the number of years he has worked and the amount of money that he has paid into Social Security per month. His work history and Social Security records will be examined to see if he meets the criteria for these categories.

An applicant for SSDI is scheduled for a medical examination to determine whether his disability is severe enough to interfere with normal work activity. If eligibility is established, SSDI benefits will be awarded retroactively to the date of application.

At the time of acceptance, a medical review date may be scheduled for the future to ascertain whether the individual's medical condition has improved sufficiently that he can rejoin the labor force. Since hemophilia is considered a permanent condition, a review date is usually not given. It is my opinion that hemophilia as a *disability* should not be considered permanent. The clinical course is variable and a mechanism for review should be included in the application. Applicants for SSDI are automatically referred to the State Department of Rehabilitation for vocational counseling. Possibly, with retraining or redirection of skills, even the most severely disabled person may be involved in work activity that is within his physical limitations.

The vocational rehabilitation counselor at the State Department of Rehabilitation receives written referrals from the Social Security Administration which include reports from the medical examinations as well as other vital data. In those cases in which it appears that vocational counseling or retraining will prepare the client for gainful employment, the counselor will contact the individual and inform him of the vocational services available to him. If the client takes advantage of these services and becomes reemployed, he can do so on a trial basis; he will continue to receive his SSDI benefits in addition to his regular paycheck for up to nine working months (these need not be consecutive). Should he find the work too strenuous, he may quit at any time during this trial period and continue to receive SSDI benefits. If he finds that he can do the work, his benefits will be discontinued three months following the end of the nine month period.

Supplementary Security Income

Someone who has little or no work history will not be eligible for SSDI because he has not made sufficient payments into the Social Security Trust Fund. This person may be eligible for Supplementary Security Income (SSI) which, as its title implies, supplements any income an individual may already receive up to a certain ceiling which is based on the cost of living. A person can receive both SSDI and SSI; that is, he may receive a small amount of SSDI benefits per month as a result of a short work history, which can be supplemented by SSI benefits.

As with SSDI, in order to be eligible for SSI, medical eligibility must be established and a medical review date scheduled unless the condition is diagnosed as permanent. Unlike SSDI, SSI may be granted almost immediately after the original medical examination since no work history records need be reviewed. There is a trial work period for SSI applicants but a large percentage of the wages are deducted from the disability payments. Once the individual is able to return to work, his SSI is immediately discontinued.

Until recently the working hemophiliac who applied for state *medical* aid on the basis of being medically indigent was liable for a share of the cost of medical expenses. This share was often unrealistically high, i.e., more than 50 percent of his income. Thus, persons with hemophilia questioned why they should work when they could avail themselves of public assistance programs and receive cash benefits and medical assistance without assuming a liability for medical expenses.

Aggressive lobbying by chapters of the National Hemophilia Foundation and their representatives has resulted in legislation in many states that provides state funds to cover the major portion of medical costs of hemophilia. Hopefully, hemophiliacs who are currently receiving public assistance such as SSI will now be motivated to seek employment.

SUMMARY

Rehabilitation counseling services have important therapeutic value in a treatment program that is designed to improve the quality of the life of the person with hemophilia. Work that the hemophilic client himself defines as meaningful is a powerful tool for developing his sense of worth and for relieving some of the tensions inherent in this chronic disease. This chapter draws on case histories and taped interviews to illustrate problems that interfere with healthy vocational development, e.g., physical limitations inherent in hemophilia, gaps and deficiencies in education, deprivation of work experience during adolescence, negative self-concept, discriminations in hiring practices, and medical indigence. The diagnosis and treatment of vocational problems require that the counselor understand the essence of the interrelationship between the biophysical, social, and psychological forces in the client's life and that he work in close collaboration with the hemophilia treatment team.

In making the vocational diagnosis, the counselor attempts to understand the hemophilic client by: (1) reconstruction of the individual's life history around major thema to provide clues to his identification model and to his life style in meeting problems, (2) psychological appraisal for insights into the way that the individual deals with interpersonal relations (a matter of first importance in vocational rehabilitation) and for indications of what the disability means to the individual in a deeply personal sense, (3) use of psychometric tests in order to match the specific trait measures of the individual with the requirements of an occupation, (4) examination of the individual's socioeconomic status and culture as an aid to understanding his attitudes towards work or a particular job, and (5) assessment of his performance in work adjustment and work evaluation activities.

Job training and placement services involve the counselor in the role of the client's advocate. To carry out the advocacy role and responsibilities, the counselor should be: (1) familiar with the general manifestations of hemophilia and its medical management, and with the patients' idiosyncratic response to the disease, (2) knowledgeable about research and demonstration findings relative to the school and employment experiences of hemophiliacs, (3) informed about workmen's compensation laws and insurance risk factors, and (4) aware of hiring practices that discriminate against the hemophiliac and of legislation that protects him.

Improved medical procedures have greatly improved the probability that hemophiliacs can carry out training programs and comply with the physical demands of their jobs. Ample training opportunities exist, as do resources for training sponsorship. Legislation designed to promote fair employment practices for persons who are handicapped will be more effective if Workmen's Compensation laws are reformed to relieve the employer of the burden of paying the full costs of compensating hemophilic workers in the event of an injury. Until recently, hemophiliacs who were working were not eligible for public aid for their medical costs unless they assumed an unrealistic share of the costs. (In order to receive full medical benefits, they had to qualify for public assistance.) Now new legislation in many states allows the working hemophiliac to qualify for state funds to pay for the major portion of the costs of medical care. Thus, hemophiliacs who are now recipients of SSI benefits should have an incentive to seek employment. Hopefully, rehabilitation counselors in public and private agencies will be serving more hemophilic clients than at any time in the past.

REFERENCES

1. Katz, A. H.: *Hemophilia: A Study in Hope and Reality.* Charles C Thomas, Springfield, 1970.
2. Taylor, C.: Educational-vocational program, in *Hemophilia: A Total Approach to Treatment and Rehabilitation.* Orthopaedic Hospital, Los Angeles, 1968.
3. Olch, D.: Effects of hemophilia upon intellectual growth and academic achievement. J. Genet. Psychol. 119:63–74, 1971.
4. Weise, P.: Sex-role identity, self-concept and vocational interests of adolescent hemophiliacs. Ph.D. Dissertation, University of Southern California, 1967.
5. Agle, D. P.: Psychiatric studies of patients with hemophilia and related studies. Arch. Intern. Med. 114:76–82, 1964.
6. Gerstein, O.: Relationship between perception of parental behavior, development of dependency, and vocational interest patterns of hemophilic young adults. Ph.D. Dissertation, New York University, 1970.
7. Kahn, E.: The impact of relationships. J. Rehabil. 38:14–17, 1972.
8. Cromwell, F.: Occupational therapy program, in *Hemophilia: A Total Approach to Treatment and Rehabilitation.* Orthopaedic Hospital, Los Angeles, 1968.
9. *Dictionary of Occupational Titles and Supplements.* U.S. Government Printing Office,

Washington, D.C., 1939 and following years.

10. *Occupational Outlook Handbook*. U.S. Government Bureau of Labor Statistics, U.S. Government Printing Office, Washington, D.C., 1949 and yearly.

11. Levine, P. H., and Britten, A. F. H.: Supervised patient-management of hemophilia: a study of forty-five patients with hemophilia A and B. Ann. Intern. Med. 78:195–201, 1973.

12. Rabiner, S. F., Telfer, M. C., and Fajardo, R.: Home transfusions of hemophiliacs. J.A.M.A. 221:885–887, 1972.

13. Lazerson, J.: Hemophilia home transfusion program: effect on school attendance. J. Pediatrics 81:330–332, 1972.

14. Taylor, C.: An exploratory study of factors associated with work injuries of hemophiliacs in Southern California, in *Hemophilia—Research, Clinical and Psycho-Social Aspects*. F. K. Schattauer-Verlag, Stuttgart, 1971.

13

FINANCIAL CONSIDERATIONS

Nancy Taylor

The provision of adequate treatment of hemophilia involves complex financial arrangements for the patient and the treatment center. Enormous expenditures of money are necessary for the treatment center to purchase the large quantities of plasma concentrates required to adequately treat a number of patients. Any hospital or medical center, public or private, will find its resources are insufficient to support a high standard of care unless most patients have adequate third party payers.

The patient may lack medical insurance coverage for a number of reasons. He may be afraid to tell his employer that he has hemophilia so he does not apply for group medical insurance available through his employer. As a child and an adolescent, he is unaware of the staggering costs of medical care because his bills have been paid by his parents' insurance or through state programs such as the Crippled Children Services. When he reaches adulthood, he may not investigate the employer's group medical insurance at the time of employment, or he considers the premiums too costly. Most group plans have open enrollment without physical examination at the time of initial employment, however, a pre-existing condition may not be covered or the insurance becomes unavailable if the application is delayed. Presently, a hemophiliac cannot purchase private insurance which adequately covers his medical costs. The hemophilic patient may easily exceed the upper limit of coverage paid through his own or his parents' insurance, although many companies have recently raised the maximum limit of coverage on group plans.

Without insurance coverage, the employed adult with average income faces constant pressure for payment of medical bills, or he does not receive adequate treatment because he cannot afford it, or he is forced to rely upon the public hospitals for his care.

The *minimal* cost for a *single* hemorrhage, based on current prices for concentrate, can easily exceed $300. For example, a man weighing 150 pounds required two infusions of six bottles of Factor VIII concentrate to arrest a hemorrhage. The cost of the concentrate was $420.00.

A federally funded program, Supplemental Security Income, provides a minimal monthly payment for living expenses while medical expenses are completely funded through the Medicaid program. Thus, many hemophilic patients must decide whether to seek employment which may or may not provide the insurance coverage or the income sufficient to pay medical expenses or to settle for state welfare with complete medical insurance. Unless he is highly skilled or extremely motivated, the decision to accept state aid can be a logical one.

FINANCIAL PLANNING

Since most patients or parents are not fully aware of third party payer resources available to them, it is essential for a treatment center to have a person available who is familiar with insurance policies and their interpretation, the constantly changing government programs and their regulations, and other possible sources of financial assistance. The institution benefits from this financial manager who is aware of patients' current financial and third party payer status and who knows when a patient needs advice and assistance. Thus, uncollectible accounts are kept at a minimum; patient anxiety and stress resulting from the presence of exceptionally large expenses can be reduced.

INVESTIGATION OF INSURANCE COVERAGE

Since a hemophiliac cannot buy adequate medical insurance privately, his usual source of insurance coverage is through a group plan sponsored by his employer or as a dependent under a parent's or a spouse's group plan.

Insurance sponsored by the employer should be investigated and an application made for it at the time of employment. Group insurance plans vary widely in their coverage. In general, those companies with greater numbers of employees in the medical insurance group will have broader coverage. Customarily, the employer pays part or all of the premium; the employee's portion is relatively inexpensive. Since insurance policies or brochures are difficult to interpret and often provide incomplete information, it is advisable to consult with someone thoroughly versed in medical insurance coverage and terminology.

Some plans do not cover blood or any blood derivatives including plasma concentrates; however, doctor visits, clinic fees, daily hospital costs, X-rays, and laboratory work will be covered. Unless the plan definitely excludes any pre-existing condition, the hemophilic employee should apply for coverage. If the hemophiliac has several job choices, he should consider the availability of adequate insurance as a prime factor in making his selection. Again, emphasis is placed upon investigating and applying for group medical insurance immediately upon employment.

Coverage of a dependent by the parent's plan varies widely and is usually extended until the dependent is 18 or 21 years old or as long as he is a full-time student. Some insurance plans offer a conversion clause so the dependent can convert the group plan to a private policy when he no longer qualifies as a dependent; however, the converted private coverage may or may not be the same as that of the group plan. The period during which conversion can occur is usually 30 days or less after the termination of dependent coverage. This conversion policy should be investigated in advance of the termination from the group plan and if treatment for hemophilia will be included under the conversion policy, application should be made without delay when the dependent reaches the stipulated age. The premiums may be expensive, but the hemophiliac should compare their expense with his average treatment costs and then determine what part of those costs would be borne by the insurance.

Insurance coverage under a spouse's group plan should be investigated immediately after marriage and application made promptly. If the wife has several job opportunities, availability of adequate insurance can be a factor in job selection. The wife may consider obtaining part-time employment to enable her husband and family to have insurance coverage.

PUBLIC ASSISTANCE PROGRAMS

Medicaid—Title XIX of the Social Security Laws, Grants to States for Medical Assistance Programs—is a public medical assistance program designed to provide necessary health care for welfare recipients and other qualified medically indigent persons or families.[1] This program is funded by state, county, and matching federal funds.

Within certain limits and guidelines, Medicaid will pay for all, or the major portion of a hemophiliac's medical treatment including inpatient hospital care, outpatient care, physicians' fees, drugs and plasma concentrates, physical therapy and dental services. The regulations and eligibilities for this program are constantly changing and vary from one geographic area to another. The county or state offices of the Department of Public Social

Services can provide information about Medicaid. These medical benefits are included as part of the Aid to Families with Dependent Children. A federal program of Supplemental Security Income for aged, blind, and disabled people with limited income and resources went into effect on January 1, 1974. In addition to a monthly cash grant, medical benefits are provided by this program. Information may be obtained from a local Social Security office.[2] Children in foster care homes, supported in whole or part by public funds, are eligible for medical care benefits. Other medically needy persons not receiving public assistance may be eligible for medical benefits under Medicaid; eligibility is determined by medical need and income. Generally, these persons are required to pay for a part of their medical expenses in the form of a calendar quarter liability with their remaining medical expenses paid under the Medicaid system. However, our experience has shown that the person's income and resources must be very low to

qualify for the program; often the liability is unrealistically high in terms of the patient's income and other expenses. Medicaid provides an opportunity for a fair hearing to any individual whose claim for medical assistance under the plan is denied or not acted upon with reasonable promptness.

Since July 1, 1973, Medicare, the two part health insurance program provided under the Social Security Administration, has been available to those patients who had been entitled to social security disability or railroad retirement disability checks for the previous 24 months.[3] The two parts of Medicare are hospital insurance and medical insurance, which will cover outpatient care. Medical coverage provided under Medicare is not as comprehensive as that under Medicaid. Outpatient coverage is provided at 80 percent under Medicare; Medicaid in most states will cover 100 percent of outpatient costs. Alabama, California, Colorado, Georgia, Illinois, Indiana, Massachusetts, Mississippi, New Jersey,

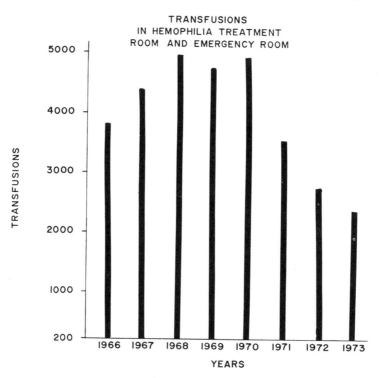

Figure 13-1. Transfusions in treatment and emergency rooms.

Ohio, Pennsylvania, South Carolina, Tennessee, and Virginia have enacted legislation providing financial assistance for medical care. Information regarding individual state programs can be obtained from chapters of the National Hemophilia Foundation.

PRIVATE SOURCES

Private sources of financing medical expenses include some of the chapters of the National Hemophilia Foundation. Contact should be made with the chapter in the patient's area to obtain information about the chapter's organization and any mechanisms for financing care. A complete listing of chapters can be obtained from the National Hemophilia Foundation, 25 West 39th St., New York, New York 10018.

INPATIENT VERSUS OUTPATIENT COSTS

As the quality and availability of outpatient care improves, both hospital admis-

sions and length of hospitalization decrease. Obviously, it is far less expensive for a patient to treat himself at home or be treated in the outpatient treatment room than to be hospitalized. As Figure 13-1 depicts, transfusions in the hemophilia treatment room and the emergency room have drastically decreased as more and more patients are treating themselves at home.

Outpatient treatment costs have ranged from over $1000 per month for several patients with severe problems to less than $100 for those with fewer bleeding episodes or with milder disease. As shown in Figure 13-2, during 1973, there were 147 hospital admissions for an average of 12 admissions per month; in 1966, there were 311 admissions for an average of 26 admissions per month.

Since plasma concentrates have become readily available, elective surgeries have steadily become more routine. In 1971 there were 21 elective surgeries, in 1972 there were 17, and in 1973 there were 26. Because of the high cost of concen-

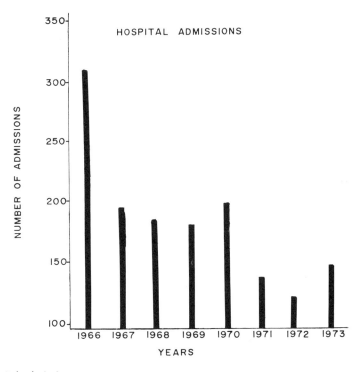

Figure 13-2. Hospital admissions.

trates, surgery for a hemophiliac is very costly. A minor surgery can cost as little as $2,500; however, it is not unusual for major procedures to cost from $16,000 to over $20,000.

Although hospital admissions have decreased since 1968, major elective surgeries with their lengthy hospitalizations have increased the number of hospital days per year as indicated in Figure 13-3. The average length of the nonsurgical hospital stay has remained essentially the same since 1968.

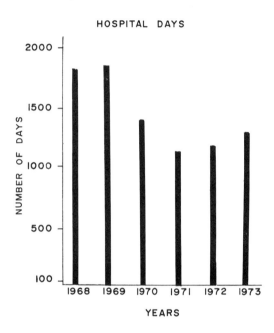

Figure 13-3. Hospital days.

MECHANISMS FOR FINANCING COSTS OF BLOOD PRODUCTS

In many areas of the United States progressive blood banks provide plasma concentrates or cryoprecipitate in exchange for donations of whole blood. Some hospital laboratories produce cryoprecipitate at a low cost. Since plasma product costs constitute the major portion of overall expenses of treatment,

such a donor mechanism effectively reduces the total burden. However, until a method is developed to provide adequate medical insurance for everyone at a reasonable cost, the problems and pressures of financing medical care for hemophiliacs will continue to exist.

It is estimated that there are 25,500 severe or moderate hemophilic patients under treatment in the United States. The estimated requirement for episodic care for these patients is 3 million whole blood units; if these patients were placed on prophylactic care, 13 million whole blood units would be required to produce the necessary plasma concentrates. However, only 9.3 million units of whole blood were collected in the United States in 1971.[4]

An additional problem exists not only in the collection of blood, but in the distribution of plasma concentrate or cryoprecipitate throughout the United States. This inadequacy is especially acute when a hemophilic patient lives in a remote area. Although many problems are evident in the collection, preparation, and distribution of blood factors, the expense of plasma products is of prime importance to the hemophiliac and his family. This situation can be alleviated somewhat by a financial manager who assists the patients in understanding the financial problems and guides them to possible sources of assistance.

REFERENCES

1. Social Security Administration, Department of Health, Education, and Welfare: *Compilation of the Social Security Laws.* 93rd Congress, 1st Session, House of Representatives, Document No. 93–117, Vol. 1.
2. U.S. Department of Health, Education, and Welfare, Social Security Administration: *Introducing Supplemental Security Income.* Publication No. (SSA) 74-11015, March 1974.
3. U.S. Department of Health, Education, and Welfare, Social Security Administration: *Your Medicare Handbook.* Baltimore, 1973.
4. National Blood Resource Program, National Institutes of Health, Department of Health, Education, and Welfare: *Pilot Study of Hemophilia Treatment in the U.S.* Bethesda, 1972.

14

HOW THE CENTER OPERATES

Donna C. Boone and Shelby L. Dietrich

As reported by the National Heart and Lung Institute in a 1972 study, 58 percent of the surveyed moderate or severe hemophiliacs in the United States received care from practitioners who treated fewer than ten hemophilic patients.[1] With so few patients, these physicians have limited opportunity to develop and to maintain proficiency in the management of hemophilia. Because of the multiple, complex problems manifested by these patients, a center for comprehensive treatment offers the best approach to provide optimum and coordinated management. A spectrum of required services is offered through specialized permanent personnel. These specialists include a hematologist with access to a coagulation laboratory, a pediatrician, an internist, an orthopedic surgeon, a physical therapist, a general dentist, an oral surgeon, a nurse with intravenous administration skills and public health orientation, a social worker, and a rehabilitation counselor. Access is highly advisable to other specialists such as a psychologist, a psychiatrist, and those in various fields of medicine and surgery.

When the staffing of a center is undertaken, the necessity for including an internist should be kept in mind. As more patients reach adulthood, the involvement of this interested specialist is essential for their total medical management. Otherwise, when patients reach adulthood, they may suddenly find themselves without comprehensive management of their chronic problems and may be reduced to receiving inadequate, sporadic care. Additionally, teenagers over age 16 or 17 may be sensitive to visiting the pediatrician and may require a direct approach to their more adult problems. All too often, the pediatrician may rely on the parent for information rather than on the patient himself; teenagers resent being ignored in this fashion and may cooperate poorly with the medical advice.

An institutional affiliation is essential; the goals of a center can only be realized in a hospital setting which includes 24 hour care with emergency room facilities under medical supervision. The supervision may be supplied by house staff who have been thoroughly oriented by regular center personnel and who have close communication with them. Inpatient and outpatient services should include a radiographic and a physical therapy department and a clinical laboratory. The center must have ready access to sufficient supplies of plasma products either through its own or a community blood bank system or through purchase of adequate stocks of pharmaceutical products. Proper center function and organization depends upon the philosophical support from hospital administration as well as a financial commitment from the hospital.

The administrative assignment of the center will vary from hospital to hospital but most often will be in the department of hematology, pediatrics, or medicine. The exact assignment does not appear to be the most crucial factor in the successful functioning of the center. However, it is critical that an interested, committed physician be in charge of the center. This specialist should realize that unilateral authoritarian decisions have no place in the total management of these patients. Obviously, immediate or life threatening medical problems must be solved by the specialist related to the problem. However, care of the chronically ill patient depends upon complete information supplied by the medical, psychological, and social team members and by the patient. Unless such a coordinated approach is utilized, the decision made unilaterally by one or two specialists may be impractical or impossible to carry out.

Irrespective of the administrative placement of the center, its director should be a member of the attending and not the house staff. The latter cannot assume the responsibility for center direction or organization because the lack of continuity of mature leadership will assure the eventual disintegration of the center. Continuity of direction is as important for the center personnel as is continuity of care for the center's patients. Indeed, this continuity of care is one of the key cornerstones in the success or failure of management of these patients and depends heavily upon the stability of the center staff.

The greatest strength of a center comes from the unity and the cohesiveness of its staff based upon mutual professional respect and demonstrated competence. Consistency of personnel is a vital factor in assuring the necessary coalescence and continuity of care. The treatment of the chronically handicapped can become distressing or burdensome to the providers of service who may become discouraged or depressed in their attempts to help these patients. At this point, staff members can provide support and guidance to each other so that the quality of professional performance remains consistently high.

Ordinarily, the majority of personnel will function only part time with the hemophilia center. Their responsibilities in the center should be clearly defined. Coordination of center activities and staff communication assumes even greater importance and becomes more difficult to achieve when staff members are present for varying periods during the work week. Regularly scheduled meetings of all the staff, including the physicians, are vital to provide a constant mechanism for staff ex-

change. The importance of these meetings cannot be overemphasized. Each staff member should feel a similar commitment for attending the meeting as he feels for visiting the patients. During these sessions, the status, the progress, and the future management of hospitalized as well as out of hospital patients can be reviewed. A systematic scrutiny of the records of all registered patients is advisable, particularly in a center with 50 or more patients. The Problem Oriented Record lends itself to this survey approach as well as to the daily notations for the active hospital record.[2,3] Thus, attention is given to all aspects of the patient's care and not solely to the most recent, acute complaint.

Attendance of staff members at the hemophilic outpatient clinics, i.e., orthopedic, pediatric, and medical, provides a further vehicle for communication and coordination of efforts. In particular this time can be appropriately utilized by the psychosocial and educational-vocational personnel for acquainting themselves with new or seldom seen patients and for initiating future appointments with those patients in need of service. In a center with 50 to 100 patients, one person can be assigned the responsibility for coordinating patient care. A physician may assume this role but more frequently the nurse specialist will be designated. Where more patients are served, various aspects of coordination may be handled by different staff members, i.e., financial matters, routine care, orthopedic aspects.

Although the genetic transmission of hemophilia A and B as sex-linked recessive traits is well known, communicating this information in a meaningful manner to patients as well as family members must become the definite responsibility of specified staff members. This information and counseling should be repeated and clarified over a period of time. Patients with von Willebrand's disease will need particular attention because of the autosomal, dominant transmission of their disease.

Inservice education of other hospital personnel involved in the direct care of hemophilic patients is important. Particularly, active, on-going training of the medical and nursing staff is vital. The staff of the center can serve as a community resource to various professional disciplines which become involved in the care or the education of the hemophilic patients. Expertise can be shared with those institutions in the formative stage of center development. Hopefully, the well established center can aid the embryonic one in avoiding some pitfalls and obstacles to providing quality care. As noted in nearly every preceding chapter, patient/parent education is the responsibility of each staff member.

The center will find itself as a referral point for evaluation of patients from outside its immediate geographic area, many of them with serious, long standing problems. Some of these patients prefer to return on a regular basis for re-evaluation of these chronic difficulties. Systematic examination by several staff members is necessary to identify all the manifestations of the problems as well as to obtain complete historical information. Here, a new patient is completely examined by the hematologist, the pediatrician or internist, the outpatient nurse, the physical therapist, the orthopedic surgeon, and the financial manager. Psychosocial and educational-vocational evaluations may be included depending upon the need and the duration of time the patient is available. Baseline laboratory examinations, including urinalysis and automated blood tests are conducted as are radiographic examinations of the chest, the pelvis, and the peripheral joints. Recommended treatment plans are subsequently formulated with and discussed with the patient, who may elect to remain at the center for the treatment.

If he is seen for evaluation only, it is important that the examination results and treatment recommendations be transmitted to the professional persons who provide his care and to the institution where he receives it. Additionally, instructions for extraordinary techniques or the use of equipment can be provided. A summary of any treatment provided at the center is important. Of particular significance is the delineation of specific follow-up care which must be carried out in the home community. Usually, it is more satisfactory if the patient can remain in the geographic

area of the center until the treatment, as originally planned, has been carried through to completion; practically, this may not be possible. However, any elective surgery should be undertaken by a center *only* when the patient can remain in the geographic area for the critical convalescent care, particularly following orthopedic procedures. Even then, thorough, careful instructions are vital for the patient and his physicians when he returns home.

Although great advances have been made in delineating the basic coagulation disorders and in the management of hemophilia in the past decade, many facets require exploration and further study. Limited financial resources and supplies of donated blood restrict the prophylactic rather than episodic care of bleeding episodes. The NHLI study of hemophilia treatment estimated that as much as 13.5 million units of whole blood would be needed to provide the plasma products which would be required for prophylaxis of the surveyed moderate and severe hemophilic patients.[1] Annual costs for such preventive care could range from 58 million to over 300 million dollars depending upon the type of plasma product used and the method by which it is produced. Advanced preparation techniques are needed to assure the greatest yield of plasma factors from each blood donation. Careful fractionation of more units of donated blood by every blood bank would increase the availability of cryoprecipitate and cryoprecipitate-poor plasma.

The precise etiology of hemarthrosis remains unclear as does the exact pathophysiologic processes which produce chronic arthropathy. Hopefully, basic investigations will not be abandoned in favor of the presently "in vogue" solutions of total joint replacement. One should avoid the overeager use of the prosthetic replacement for this particular group of younger aged, active patients with their present and potential involvement of multiple peripheral joints, especially weight bearing ones.

The current challenge of chronic pain management coupled with drug abuse or misuse appears to increase in magnitude as more patients reach young and middle adulthood. The extent of the problem is unclear for the hemophilic population as well as in comparison with drug abuse/misuse statistics from other diseased groups with chronic pain manifestations and the nondiseased general population.

The approaches to the management of tension, emotional stress, and pain should be expanded beyond the traditional drug prescription to include the exploration of introspective techniques such as biofeedback, autosuggestion, and transcendental meditation. Although our experiences with group psychotherapy have been limited and generally unsatisfactory, this treatment vehicle should be examined further. However, the group's therapist should anticipate some inconsistency in attendance of the group members due to bleeding episodes and other factors. Increased participation of psychologists and psychiatrists as staff members of hemophilia centers is expected and should be encouraged. As the past few years can be described as "the days of the hematologists," perhaps, during the next decade, the psychosocial disciplines will have "their turn at the wheel."

Life expectancy figures need study and probable revision since the advent of plasma concentrates and improved methods of medical treatment. Up to date actuarial data may aid hemophilic patients in obtaining life and other insurance. Additionally, a retrospective review of the causes of mortality of hemophiliacs may reveal those deaths which were preventable as well as those with social or psychiatric implications. Systematic scrutiny on a prospective basis should be instituted.

Further exploration should be made of the vocational selection process and problems encountered by hemophilic persons. Comparisons with previous studies related to work selection, employment and unemployment status as well as work stability and absenteeism appear necessary in view of the decade interval since these facets were surveyed.[4,5] Additional analysis of the relation of achievement level to the tested behavior and intelligence of these patients should be explored more completely. As

illustrated by the following case history, identification of those crucial ingredients which turn a person with many "strikes against him" into a productive society member is elusive:

This black man was initially seen at this Center in 1968 at 19 years of age. A diagnosis of severe Factor VIII deficiency with *high titer inhibitor* was confirmed. By history, his childhood and adolescence were replete with multiple bleeding episodes for which he received whole blood and/or plasma. Hospitalizations were frequent.

During the six years of his treatment at this Center, he was hospitalized a total of 86 days for management of multiple soft tissue hemorrhages, repeated shoulder hemarthrosis, hematuria, and abdominal pain and vomiting secondary to acute and chronic cholecystitis with cholelithiasis. Severe caries were found which necessitated restorative and surgical dental management. Joint limitation and degenerative arthritic changes were evident in the shoulders, knees, and ankles. Routine outpatient management of joint and peripheral soft tissue hemorrhages consisted of analgesics and short-term steroid therapy. Radiation therapy was administered to attempt to reduce the marked, disabling bilateral shoulder pain secondary to severe degeneration.

His educational background indicated that he had always attended schools for the handicapped; school absences were chronic problems. He "dropped out" of school in his senior year of high school because of frequent, prolonged absences. When initially evaluated here, he scored in the average range of intelligence on the Wechsler Adult Intelligence Scale with slightly higher scores on performance than on verbal ability. His scores on the Wide Range Achievement test placed him at junior high school levels even though he had been placed in the senior class.

His previous work experience included three short-term, part time jobs: grocery store clerk, service station and snack bar attendant. All were too difficult for his physical abilities. A referral was made for him to the Department of Rehabilitation with their subsequent sponsorship of a ten week course in electronic production; the course included instruction in reading diagrams and blueprints as well as wiring and soldering computer components.

Following his electronic training, he worked for seven months for an electronic production company; he was terminated at the end of the company's subcontract. He found subsequent employment in a similar company for a four month period until the company went bankrupt. He could not obtain further employment in the depressed electronics field so with Center staff encouragement, he decided to return to school at an occupational center where he was able to complete credits for his high school diploma and to receive training as a hospital ward clerk. The Department of Rehabilitation sponsored this training, also. Currently, he is employed as a ward clerk and although he enjoys this work, he plans to continue his education toward the goal of becoming an inhalation therapist.

He recently stated, "It feels good to be working and contributing to society particularly in the hospital area where so much has been done for me!"

If only we could discover what forces have motivated this young man to persevere in his attempts to become a "giver" to society rather than a "taker" in spite of the severe racial, cultural, educational, and medical obstacles facing him.

REFERENCES

1. National Heart Lung Institute: *Pilot Study of Hemophilia Treatment in the United States.* Blood Resource Studies, Vol. 3, National Institutes of Health, Department of Health, Education, and Welfare, Bethesda, 1972.
2. Weed, L. L.: *Medical Records, Medical Education, and Patient Care.* The Press of Case Western Reserve University, Cleveland, 1969.
3. Hurst, J. W., and Walker, H. K.: *The Problem-Oriented System.* Medcom Press, New York, 1972.
4. Taylor, C.: Educational-Vocational Program, in *Hemophilia: A Total Approach to Treatment and Rehabilitation.* Orthopaedic Hospital, Los Angeles, 1968.
5. Katz, A. H.: *Hemophilia. A Study in Hope and Reality.* Charles C Thomas, Publisher, Springfield, 1970.

APPENDICES

APPENDIX 1

ADMINISTRATION OF PLASMA PRODUCTS

PREPARATION OF CRYOPRECIPITATE AND FRESH FROZEN PLASMA

These products are stored at −30° C. Prior to administration, they are thawed in a water bath at 37° C or less. Always check the temperature with a thermometer since hotter water will destroy Factor VIII. Both cryoprecipitate and fresh frozen plasma must be administered within one hour after removal from the freezer. Factor VIII deteriorates when the thawed products remain at room temperature for extended periods of time. When a patient must receive 15 or more bags of cryoprecipitate in one infusion, one half of the required number of bags are thawed and the infusion is started. Then, the remaining bags are thawed and administered.

Cryoprecipitate is used for treatment of:

1. Hemophilia A
2. Von Willebrand's disease

Fresh frozen plasma is used for treatment of:
1. Mild hemophilia A or B
2. Von Willebrand's disease
3. Patients with undiagnosed bleeding problems

PREPARATION OF FACTOR VIII AND FACTOR IX CONCENTRATE

Concentrates are stored at 2 to 8°C. They are never stored below freezing. Ever increasing numbers of plasma concentrates are being manufactured by pharmaceutical companies. Basically, all the products are prepared for administration by the same technique. However, the manufacturer's instructions should be carefully followed. *Each concentrate is specifically manufactured for one type of hemophilia.*

The concentrate should always be reconstituted with the solution, sterile water or normal saline, provided by the manufacturer. Water should not be substituted for saline nor saline for water. Diluents containing preservatives should never be used.

The diluent *should not be warmed* to a temperature over 37° C since a hot solution will reduce the potency of Factor VIII. Additionally, the lyophilized material will not dissolve completely when too warm and cannot be administered.

Concentrates which are prepared with small volumes of diluent (10 cc or less) are administered through a syringe. Reconstituted concentrate from several bottles can be drawn into a 50 cc syringe for administration. Large volumes of dissolved concentrate (25 cc or more per bottle) are administered through intravenous tubing, which is usually supplied by the manufacturer.

Administration of these concentrates is based upon complete diagnosis of the type and severity of hemophilia: (1) Factor VIII (AHF) concentrate is used *only* for treatment of severe or moderate hemophilia A. (2) Factor IX (PTC) concentrate is used for treatment of severe hemophilia B. Patients with moderate hemophilia B may use Factor IX concentrate or fresh frozen plasma.

CHOICE OF VEINS

Upper Extremity

First choices: venous cephalica and venous basilica between the antecubital fossa and wrist.

Alternative: Dorsal venous plexus. These veins have a tendency to "roll;" their puncture should be attempted only by a highly skilled nurse or physician.

Lower Extremity

Dorsal venous plexus: These veins may be used on an infant, if upper extremity veins are unsuitable. However, older patients complain that venipuncture at these sites is painful.

It is advisable not to use the small, superficial veins of the volar surface of the wrist because infiltration of the concentrate into surrounding tissues occurs easily. Severe swelling and pain may result with subsequent compression of neurovascular structures leading to impaired function of the hand. These veins are so small that the concentrate is not diluted with sufficient venous blood. As a result, the patient frequently complains of stinging and burning along the path of the vein, proximal to the venipuncture.

Frequently used veins may become inflamed or thickly scarred and painful. When repetitive dosages of concentrate are administered over a short time interval, a different vein should be selected for each infusion.

NEEDLE SELECTION

Needles larger than 20 gauge cause greater trauma and scarring of veins than do small ones and should be used only during blood transfusions or surgery. Some plastic intravenous catheters are suspected of contributing to phlebitis. When concentrates are administered (especially Factor IX) in combination with a plastic cannula, careful observation of the limb is essential. The cannula should be replaced by a needle at the first sign of inflammation or if the patient complains of pain along the vein proximal to the cannula.

To administer concentrate or cryoprecipitate to infants and toddlers, the needle of choice is a 22 or 23 gauge scalp vein needle. (Deseret Minicath or Abbott Butterfly.) For older children and adults, a 21 gauge scalp vein or one inch straight needle is used. A size 20 gauge needle may be used to obtain blood specimens for laboratory tests.

RATE OF ADMINISTRATION OF SOLUTION

When plasma products are administered with a drip set and a size 21 gauge or smaller needle, the clamp on the tubing can be fully open. Concentrate administered by syringe may be injected no faster than 1 ml per four to five seconds.

REACTIONS TO CONCENTRATE

If the patient complains of dizziness, tingling around the mouth, headache, nausea, or if his face appears flushed, the rate of infusion is slowed. If the symptoms persist or increase in severity, infusion of the concentrate is stopped; other acceptable solution is administered through a separate tubing to maintain an "open" I.V.; the physician is notified. Allergic reactions such as severe hives or bronchial spasm are more usual during infusion of cryoprecipitate or plasma but can occur during concentrate administration. Antihistamines and adrenalin are available for the physician to administer if symptoms persist or increase in severity.

Patients with a prior history of allergic reactions are given oral antihistamines one half hour prior to all infusions.

REACTIONS TO CRYOPRECIPITATE OR PLASMA

Allergic reactions, including hives, are not uncommon when cryoprecipitate or plasma is infused. If reactions occur, diphenhydramine hydrochloride (Benadryl) or other antihistamine is administered intravenously by a Center physician or the nurse. These patients receive oral Benadryl one half hour prior to any future infusions of cryoprecipitate or plasma. Cryoprecipitate is not given to the few patients who develop extreme allergic response to it. Concentrate is used instead. Rarely, severe hives, flushing, nausea, bronchial spasm, or headache occurs. When this happens, an acceptable solution such as normal saline is administered through separate tubing to maintain an "open" I.V. The infusion of cryoprecipitate or plasma is stopped and a physician is contacted *immediately*.

INFILTRATION OF SOLUTION

If the patient complains of stinging at the site of venipuncture, the solution may be infiltrating. Swelling may be observed at site of venipuncture. It is usually advisable to discontinue the infusion and select another vein.

DISCONTINUING THE INFUSION

Pressure is not applied over the vein until the needle is completely removed; otherwise, the posterior wall of the vein may be lacerated. Firm, steady pressure for one or two minutes will usually halt bleeding. The area is not massaged since this manipulation may dislodge the formed clot and cause a hematoma to form. Finally, a small adhesive bandage, or occasionally a small pressure dressing, is applied. The latter is used following venipuncture of the lower extremity.

APPENDIX 2

HOME TRANSFUSION INSTRUCTIONS

DOSAGE INSTRUCTIONS

Name _____ Date _____
Weight _____

Dosages of Factor VIII and Factor IX concentrates are based upon the body weight of the patient, the severity of the hemophilia, and severity of the hemorrhages. Changes in weight may necessitate recalculation of dosages.

The number of units of clotting factor per bottle varies greatly; therefore, always calculate the dose very carefully. Factor VIII is the antihemophilic factor (AHF) which is the clotting factor missing in hemophilia A (classic hemophilia). Factor IX is the plasma thromboplastin component (PTC) and is the clotting factor missing in patients who suffer from hemophilia B (Christmas disease).

There is always a danger of contacting hepatitis when handling these plasma concentrates. If a family member, who is assisting with the administration procedures, accidentally stabs himself with a used needle, he should promote bleeding of the stab wound and wash the area thoroughly with soap and water. Skin to mouth contact with spilled concentrate also poses a hepatitis source. Therefore, on completion of the procedure, anyone who handled the concentrate should wash his hands thoroughly. The work area should also be cleaned after safe disposal of used equipment, i.e., place all used needles and syringes in a closed container.

These instructions are to be followed explicitly. If you have any problems, doubts, or questions regarding management of a hemorrhage, do not hesitate to call the Center nurse.

The concentrate dose may be repeated in 24 hours if a minor hemorrhage has not resolved. If, after a second dose of concentrate has been administered, the hemorrhage fails to resolve, contact the Center nurse. *If you sustain a severe injury or are involved in an automobile accident,* contact the Center nurse or physician immediately. The telephone number for all calls is 747-4481, extension 441 or 436.

Area of Bleeding	*Desired Factor Level*	*# Units*
1. Minor or moderate *knee, elbow, ankle, shoulder, wrist.*	30%	_____
2. Severe *knee, elbow, ankle, shoulder, wrist. If joint is* very swollen and painful, *do not* give concentrate. Come to Center or Emergency Room for aspiration. Concentrate will be given at the time of aspiration.	50%	_____
3. *Hip* or *retroperitoneal* hemorrhages (may not be able to differentiate) or any hemorrhage in which groin area pain and hip and/or knee flexion are evident, call Hemophilia Center nurse when this occurs. Do not bear weight on affected leg.	50%	_____

4. Minor or moderate *calf* or *forearm* hemorrhage.	30%	_____
5. Severe *forearm* hemorrhages. Call Hemophilia Center nurse immediately or come to clinic or Emergency Room. A forearm hemorrhage may require a plaster molded splint.	50%	_____
6. For a severe *calf* or *popliteal* (in back of knee) hemorrhage. Call Center nurse. Do not bear any weight on affected leg until advised to by Center physician.	50%	_____
7. *Soft tissue* and *muscle* hemorrhages of minor or moderate severity, e.g., thigh, buttock, back, upper arm.	30%	_____
8. Severe *soft tissue* or *muscle* hemorrhages (buttock, thigh, back, upper arm). Call Center nurse or come to clinic or Emergency Room.	50%	_____
9. *Abdominal* or *chest wall* hemorrhages. Call Center nurse or come immediately to the hospital if there is more than minor discomfort.	50%	_____
10. *Gastrointestinal* bleeding (vomiting blood, bleeding through rectum, or black, tarry stools). Call or come to the Center or Emergency Room immediately.	50%	_____
11. *Spitting* or *coughing up blood. Do not give concentrate.* Come immediately to Center or Emergency Room.		
12. *Head injuries.* COME IMMEDIATELY TO CENTER OR EMERGENCY ROOM WHETHER OR NOT SIGNS OF HEMORRHAGE ARE EVIDENT. Give concentrate at home unless you are anxious about possible severe injury. It is very important to come to the hospital. Do not drive yourself. Contact family member or neighbor or call an ambulance.	50%	_____
13. *Neck* or *throat* hemorrhage. Call Center nurse. If there is any difficulty in swallowing or breathing come to Center immediately.	50%	_____
14. *Urinary bleeding.* Increase fluid intake to one glass every hour and one glass every two hours at night. Call Center nurse.	50%	_____
15. *Gum, tongue, lip, mouth, or nose* bleeding. It is necessary to repeat this dose every 24 hours for 2 to 3 days even though bleeding has stopped. Any large strawberry like clots should be removed from the mouth following concentrate administration.	30%	_____
16. *Prophylactic dose* (to prevent bleeding)	20–30%	_____

PREPARATION AND ADMINISTRATION OF FACTOR VIII AND FACTOR IX CONCENTRATES

Collect the prescribed number of bottles of the right concentrate together with the diluent which is supplied by the manufacturer. Some concentrates are reconstituted with sterile water and others with normal saline. Always use the diluent supplied with the specific concentrate. Never reconstitute concentrate with a diluent containing preservatives. Factor VIII concentrates are used specifically for patients with AHF deficiency hemophilia (classic hemophilia, hemophilia A). Factor IX concentrates are used for patients with Factor IX deficiency hemophilia (Christmas disease, hemophilia B).

Syringe Method

Equipment

1. Prescribed number of concentrate and diluent bottles.
2. Plastic disposable syringe. Do not use glass syringes. The size of the syringe depends on the volume of concentrate to be administered.
3. Filter needle if the manufacturer requires the concentrate to be filtered.
4. Size 18, 20, or 21 needle.
5. Size 21 or 23 scalp vein or minicath needle.
6. Tourniquet.
7. Alcohol sponges.
8. Dry cotton ball.
9. Band-Aid.

Procedure for Administration

1. Have all equipment on hand.
2. Wash hands thoroughly with soap and water.
3. Remove caps from diluent and concentrate bottles.
4. Swab the exposed rubber stoppers with alcohol sponges. Do not leave excess alcohol on the rubber.
5. Remove water from the first diluent bottle using the plastic syringe with a size 18, 20, or 21 needle attached.
6. Inject this water gently into the dried concentrate. Direct the stream of water toward the side of the bottle to avoid forming excess foam in the bottle.
7. Repeat this procedure for all bottles to be administered.
8. Agitate all bottles *gently* or rotate concentrate bottle until all concentrate is dissolved. Do not shake vigorously. If, after agitating for 10 or 15 minutes, you find some "stubborn" lumps that won't dissolve, place the concentrate bottles in a bath of water warmed to *98.6° F* for a few minutes, then remove and continue agitating. The warm water bath helps dissolve the lumps. Always use a thermometer to check the temperature of the water bath. Water that is over 98.6° F will destroy the potency of the concentrate.
9. When the concentrate has dissolved, wipe the rubber stoppers with a damp alcohol sponge.
10. Attach filter needle to plastic syringe.
11. Withdraw contents of reconstituted bottles into syringes.
12. Remove filter needle.
13. Attach scalp vein needle to syringe. Size 21 is adequate for most people. If the veins are very small, you may prefer a size 23.
14. Fill scalp vein tubing with concentrate. Do not spill concentrate. It is best to leave the last inch or so of the tubing empty.
15. Assume a comfortable position with a pillow supporting the extremity of proposed transfusion site.
16. Apply tourniquet at least three inches above site where you plan to insert needle.
17. Wipe area of proposed infusion site vigorously with an alcohol sponge.
18. Insert needle. If needle is in vein, blood will return immediately. Remove tourniquet.
19. Administer concentrate at the rate of 1 cc every three to five seconds. If you experience dizziness or tingling around the mouth, slow the infusion.
20. When the infusion is finished, remove needle.
21. Apply firm, steady pressure for two or three minutes at the infusion site. Do not massage.
22. Apply Band-Aid.
23. Complete log of transfusion.

Drip Method

Equipment

1. The prescribed number of concentrate and diluent bottles.
2. Plastic tubing (comes with concentrate).
3. Airways (comes with tubing).
4. Double-ended needles (comes with tubing).
5. Tape, one inch; "paper" tape is preferable.
6. Needles, preferably one inch, size 21 or size 21 scalp vein.

7. Tourniquet.

8. Alcohol sponges.

9. Dry cotton balls.

10. Band-Aid.

11. Hook on which to hang the concentrate placed above head of person receiving concentrate.

12. 20 cc plastic disposable syringe.

Procedure for Administration

1. Have all equipment on hand.

2. Wash hands thoroughly with soap and water.

3. Remove aluminum bands and dust cap from the diluent and concentrate bottles.

4. Swab the exposed rubber surfaces with alcohol sponges. Do not leave excess alcohol on the rubber surfaces.

5. Take the double-ended needle. Remove one end of the covering. Do not touch needle.

6. Insert this exposed end of the double-ended needle through the depression in the center of the stopper in the bottle of diluent.

7. Remove covering from the other end of the double-ended needle.

8. Invert diluent bottle directly over the concentrate bottle so that the rubber stoppers from each bottle are facing each other.

9. Push the exposed end of the double-ended needle into the depression in the center of the concentrate bottle. There should be enough vacuum to draw all the water into the concentrate.

   a. If the water will not be drawn into the concentrate bottle, remove the double-ended needle from the concentrate bottle and reinsert.

   b. If the vacuum is lost and the water will not go into the concentrate bottle, you may need to withdraw the water into the 20 cc disposable syringe and inject it into the concentrate. When injecting 20 cc of water into the concentrate bottle, be sure to remove 20 cc of air before removing syringe. This is very important as it relieves pressure in concentrate bottle.

   c. Be sure that the needle in the diluent bottle is always below the level of the water.

10. When all the water has been drawn into the concentrate, disconnect the two bottles by withdrawing the needle from the concentrate bottle.

11. Use one double-ended needle for all bottles of concentrate. After withdrawing the double-ended needle from the first bottle of concentrate, insert that end into the next diluent (water) bottle; then withdraw the other end from the old (the one that has already been used) diluent bottle and insert that end of the needle into the next bottle of concentrate. Be sure that the diluent bottle is inverted directly over the concentrate. Be careful not to touch the needle portions; hold double-ended needle only by middle section. Repeat this procedure until all bottles are mixed. If any needle is contaminated by touching, discard it and use a new needle.

12. Agitate or rotate all concentrate bottles *gently* until all concentrate is dissolved. Do not shake vigorously. If after agitating for 10 or 15 minutes you find some "stubborn" lumps that won't dissolve, place the concentrate bottles in a bath of water warmed to 98.6° F for a few minutes. Then remove and continue agitating. The warm water bath helps dissolve the lumps. Always use a thermometer to check the temperature of the water bath. Water that is over 98.6° F will destroy the potency of the concentrate.

13. When the concentrate has dissolved, wipe the rubber stoppers with a damp alcohol sponge. The rubber stopper on some types of concentrate contains a small depression specifically for an air vent needle. If this is so, insert the air vent needle all the way in. Other bottles have only one depression in the center. If this is so, insert the air vent needle to one side of the depression and push the needle diagonally toward the center of the bottle. Be sure to insert the needle all the way into the bottle. If there is a piece of cotton in the hub of the air vent needle, remove it.

14. If you have bottle jackets, place one on each bottle. If you do not, you can make them by cutting a piece of adhesive tape about 4 inches long. Fold the tape in

half, sticky side inside, except for the ends. Place the ends on opposite sides of the bottom sides of concentrate bottles so that the tape looks like a basket handle. Take another piece of tape about 4 inches long and wrap it around the bottle to secure the ends of the first piece of tape.

15. Hold the tubing and close the clamp.

16. Remove cover from stopper-puncture needle of set (near the drip chamber) and insert this needle into the depression in the concentrate bottle stopper. Suspend the bottle upside down from a wall hook.

17. Squeeze and release the drip chamber about two or three times to allow it to fill partially with liquid.

18. Open the control clamp and fill the tubing with liquid from the concentrate bottles. As soon as the tubing is filled, close the clamp. Do not waste concentrate.

19. Remove the plastic covering from the end of the tubing. Place the needle or scalp vein needle that you will insert into the vein on the end of the tubing. The concentrate and tubing are now ready for administration.

20. Cut three strips of tape three inches long; place them where you will be able to reach them easily.

21. Sit in a comfortable chair where adequate lighting is available. Place a pillow under the arm which will be used to start the infusion.

22. Apply tourniquet about three inches above site of proposed needle insertion.

23. Make a fist if an arm vein is being used. With the index finger from the other hand, feel the direction of the vein so that you will know which way to insert the needle.

24. When you are sure you know where you will insert the needle, wipe the area with an alcohol sponge.

25. Insert needle with bevel up (sharp point down so this sharp point will puncture the skin first). Insert it very slowly and carefully. When the needle is in the vein you will see a blood return in the tubing. Release the tourniquet and

then the clamp without disturbing the position of the needle in the vein. If you have assistance, another person can release the clamp. If you use a scalp vein needle, you will have a fairly good blood return when the needle is correctly in the vein. If you use a straight needle, a small blood return will be noted. If in doubt, pinch and release the tubing next to the needle, or lower the bottle and open the clamp to check. If there is little or no blood return, the needle may have gone through the vein into the surrounding tissues.

26. When needle is in the vein:

    a. Tape needle in place.

    b. Hang bottle with other hand.

The infusion should be running well. If it is not, check the following:

    a. Be sure the clamp is completely open.

    b. Be sure the tourniquet has been removed.

    c. Place a small square of alcohol sponge directly beneath the tubing near the point where the vein needle fits into the tubing, or rotate needle slightly. This will change the position of the needle in the vein.

    d. Squeeze the drip chamber.

    e. Be sure the airway is not plugged with cotton.

27. If the infusion will not run after adjusting and manipulating, it may be necessary to discontinue and restart it. If a burning sensation is felt around the site of needle entry, this is an indication that the concentrate is infiltrating (going) into the tissue surrounding the vein. Discontinue it immediately.

28. Assuming that the infusion is going well:

    a. Clamp the tubing after first bottle has emptied into it.

    b. Remove airway from first bottle and insert it into second bottle.

    c. Remove stopper-puncture needle from first bottle and insert it into second bottle.

    d. Hang the second bottle on the hook.

    e. Release clamp. When you become skilled at changing the needles between bottles, you need not clamp the tubing each time.

29. When the concentrate from the last bottle has entered the tubing, disconnect the tubing from the bottle. Fold the tubing between the drip chamber and the stopper-puncture needle. Simultaneously, squeeze the drip chamber. Repeat this until all concentrate is squeezed into the vein. Be sure to stop squeezing before you push air into the vein.

30. Clamp the tubing immediately when all the concentrate is in vein.

31. Remove tape carefully.

32. Remove needle from vein.

33. Apply steady, firm pressure to puncture site with a dry cotton ball for two to three minutes. DO NOT MASSAGE.

34. Do not apply pressure as you withdraw the needle.

35. Apply Band-Aid.

36. Complete log of transfusions.

APPENDIX 3

THE ANTERIOR OPENED-THIGH THERMOPLASTIC SPLINT

The anterior opened-thigh thermoplastic splint is used to immobilize the knee following hemarthrosis with marked pain and swelling; to support during walking whenever muscle strength is inadequate to properly protect the knee; and to retain a corrected position of knee extension following removal of the extension desubluxation hinge and the opened-thigh nonremovable cylinder casts.

The following materials are required: a large sheet of paper for preparing pattern, tubular stockinette, masking or paper tape, a sheet (or sheets) of thermoplastic material, 4 inch elastic bandages, heavy duty scissors, professional contact cement (obtained from a hardware store), thermoplastic cement, Velcro hook and pile in 1 inch widths.

Fabricating the Posterior Portion

1. Place sheet of paper beneath leg to extend from heel to buttocks.
2. Trace outline of the posterior two thirds of the leg on the paper by positioning the medial and lateral portions of the paper close to the leg (Fig. 1).

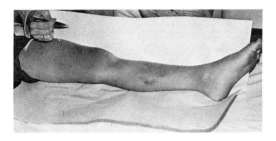

Figure 1.

3. Cut out the pattern which extends from just below the buttock to the level of the malleoli (Fig. 2).

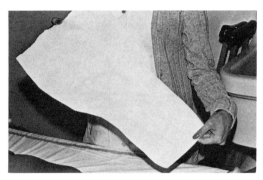

Figure 2.

4. Position the pattern about the posterior aspect of the leg and mark the pattern to more exactly conform to the leg. Allow sufficient space about the knee to avoid compressing the patella (Fig. 3).

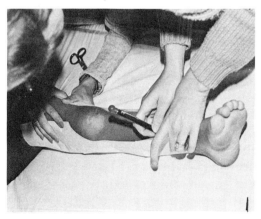

Figure 3.

165

5. Trim the pattern accordingly and crease areas for better contour; tape the creased areas (Fig. 4 and 5).

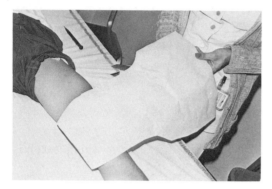

Figure 4.

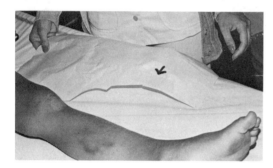

Figure 5.

6. Check the fit of the pattern again.
7. Trace an outline of the refitted pattern on a sheet of thermoplastic material (Fig. 6).

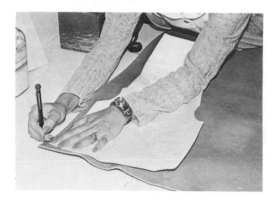

Figure 6.

8. Submerge the thermoplastic into a hydrocollator pack machine (or a large flat pan of 140° F water) to soften the material and expedite cutting it (Fig. 7).

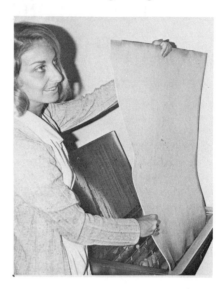

Figure 7.

9. Cut the thermoplastic with heavy duty scissors following the traced outline. Contour all corners (Fig. 8).

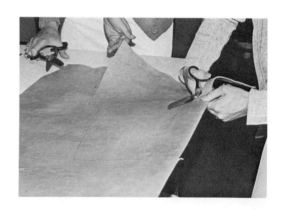

Figure 8.

10. Submerge the cut thermoplastic into the hot water for several minutes to thoroughly soften.
11. Place a length of tubular stockinette on the patient's leg from foot to buttock (Fig. 9).

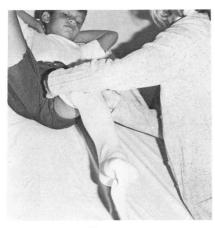

Figure 9.

12. Remove softened thermoplastic from the water and dry with towels to absorb all the hot water (Fig. 10).

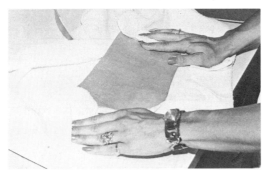

Figure 10.

13. Mold thermoplastic to the leg with the knee in maximum extension with one person maintaining the position of the thermoplastic close to the contour of the leg and the other person rolling elastic bandages tightly around the leg and the thermoplastic (Fig. 11).

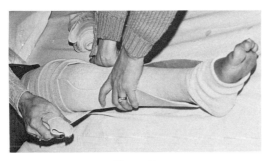

Figure 11.

14. Maintain the elastic wrapping over the thermoplastic for at least 30 minutes for the material to become rigid.

15. If extra support is needed for a large patient, ⅜ inch strips (ribs) of thermoplastic may be applied longitudinally using thermoplastic cement after the posterior portion becomes rigid. Further support can be obtained with a double thickness of the thermoplastic. Two pieces of material are traced and cut in steps 7 through 9. The second piece is molded and adhered with thermoplastic cement to the posterior section after the first has hardened. Additional time is required for the second piece to become rigid.

Fabricating the Anterior Portion

16. Remove the elastic bandages from the posterior portion and with that portion still on the leg, trace and fit a paper pattern to cover the anterior lower leg from the level of the malleoli to the level of the tibial plateau and extending over the sides of the posterior portion of the splint (Fig. 12).

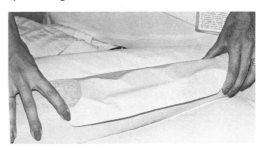

Figure 12.

17. Trace the outline of the anterior portion onto the thermoplastic (Fig. 13).

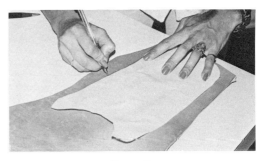

Figure 13.

18. Cut and soften the thermoplastic as previously described.

19. Apply the anterior portion overlapping the posterior portion still in position. Wrap the entire leg with elastic bandages (Fig. 14).

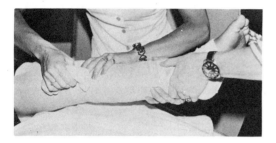

Figure 14.

20. When the anterior and posterior sections are rigid, two strips of Velcro hook are attached with the contact cement to the anterior portion and the lower leg portion of the posterior. Long straps of Velcro pile are wrapped about the hook to maintain the position of the splint (Fig. 15).

Adjusting the Splint

21. Soften the portion requiring adjustment with a hair dryer or in a pan of 140° F water.

22. Slightly cool and dry the material with toweling if water was used; place the splint on the leg while the material is soft

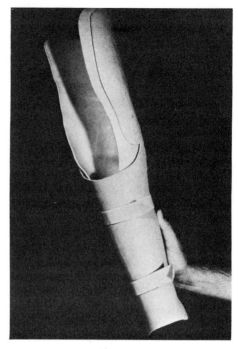

Figure 15.

and warm. Wrap the elastic bandages as shown in the previous instructions.

23. Allow the thermoplastic to harden for 30 to 40 minutes before removing the elastic bandages.

24. Foam rubber padding (¼ inch to ½ inch in width) may be placed inside the bottom edge of the splint if irritation occurs about the ankle. Additionally, the thermoplastic may be flared outward to reduce malleoli and heel cord pressure.

APPENDIX 4
THE EXTENSION DESUBLUXATION HINGE CAST

When chronic problems of severe knee joint restriction, tibial subluxation, and moderate to severe degenerative changes are present, extension desubluxation hinges are used to gradually extend the knee and to attempt to desublux the tibia. Maximum correction from one casting will be obtained in a two to three week period or less. Correction beyond 10 to 15 degrees flexion is not obtained usually. An anterior opened-thigh cylinder cast or thermoplastic splint is used to retain this corrected position. In some patients with severe degeneration, marked joint pain or discomfort may occur during the casting period; administration of analgesic medication may be necessary. When the hinges are used on hemophilic patients, prophylactic infusion of plasma products, of the appropriate type and dosage, prior to the application will eliminate the chances of hemorrhage secondary to the procedure. Additional dosages of plasma products are used only if any bleeding episodes become evident; these are rare.

These hinges were designed by G. Carlton Wallace, M.D. for hemophilic patients during his resident training period at Orthopaedic Hospital. Modifications of the design were made subsequently by William A. Craig, M.D. California Design and Manufacturing Company, 1732 Tanen St., Napa, California 94558 is the manufacturer and supplier.

Application of the Extension Desubluxation Hinges

1. Take radiographs and range of motion measurements of the knee prior to casting (Fig. 1).

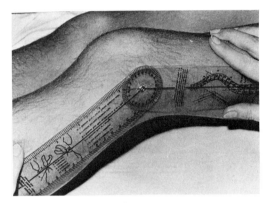

Figure 1.

2. Position the supine patient with the involved knee in maximum comfortable extension for the casting procedure.

3. Place two sections of tubular stockinette on the leg: an upper thigh portion and a lower calf portion; the area about the knee is exposed (Fig. 2).

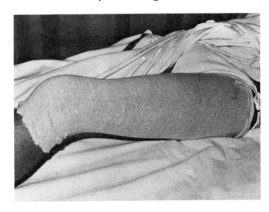

Figure 2.

4. Elevate the foot on a casting block with the knee in extension (Fig. 3).

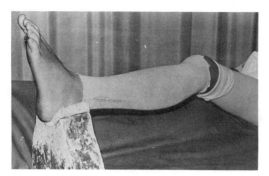

Figure 3.

5. Mark position of the knee joint line on the skin medially and laterally.

Ankle-to-Knee Portion

6. Wrap cotton soft roll or sheet wadding from ankle to knee (Fig. 4).

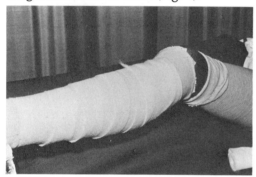

Figure 4.

7. Place a 1½ to 2 inch strip of adhesive foam (such as Spenco Skin Guard) over the stockinette above the malleoli as well as distal to the patella at the point of pressure over the tibia (Fig. 5).

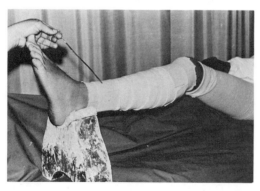

Figure 5.

8. Wrap soft roll or sheet wadding over the adhesive foam.

9. Apply one 4 inch or 6 inch roll of plaster over the soft roll from ankle to knee (Fig. 6).

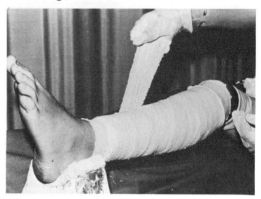

Figure 6.

10. Turn back stockinette over plaster after first roll has been applied to make a cushion of the double thickness of foam rubber and apply second roll of plaster. Form fit the cylinder by molding well.

Knee-to-Hip Portion

11. Wrap soft roll or sheet wadding from knee to upper thigh (Fig. 7).

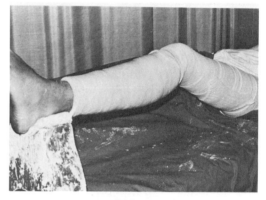

Figure 7.

12. Trim a one half inch foam rubber pad to conform to patellar area and to cover the patellar area and the lower portion of the quadriceps. Bevel the edges of the pad.

13. Place foam pad over patellar-distal

quadriceps area and place a 2 inch strip of adhesive foam circumferentially at the proximal thigh (Fig. 8).

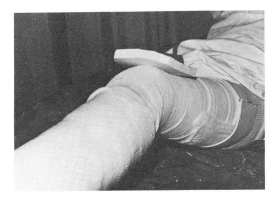

Figure 8.

14. Wrap soft roll over the foam to anchor in place.

15. Apply one 4 inch or 6 inch roll of plaster from the knee to the upper thigh.

16. Apply two 4″ × 15″ plaster splints (three thicknesses each) longitudinally to sponge rubber patellar extension to reinforce it (Fig. 9).

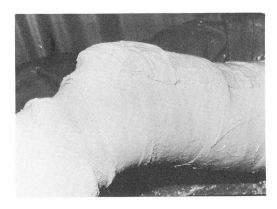

Figure 9.

17. Turn stockinette over plaster and apply second roll of plaster (Fig. 10). Form fit the thigh cylinder very carefully by molding the plaster.

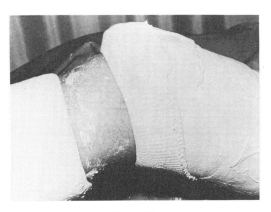

Figure 10.

Applying the Hinges

18. Apply the hinges with knee in comfortable extension (Fig. 11).

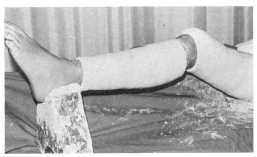

Figure 11.

19. Adjust the screws of the hinges to allow the greatest amount of correction as they are turned.

20. Adjust the left hinge for the left side of the knee (Fig. 12) and the right hinge for the right side of the knee (Fig. 13).

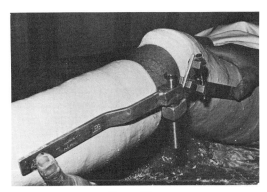

Figure 12.

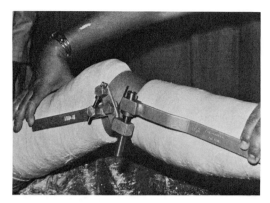

Figure 13.

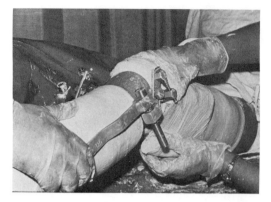

Figure 15.

21. Apply the hinges with the axis (Fig. 14) aligned with the marked joint line; the flexion correction screw is proximal to the knee joint; the desubluxing screw is distal to the knee joint and essentially perpendicular to the tibia.

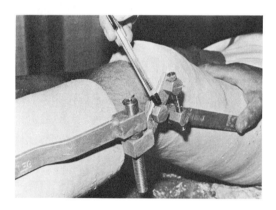

Figure 14.

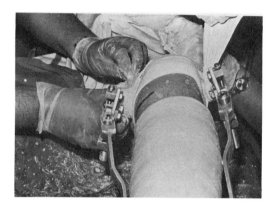

Figure 16.

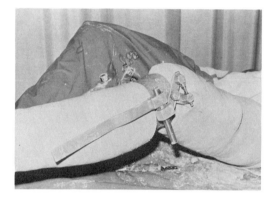

Figure 17.

22. Apply the hinges as nearly parallel as possible. Bending irons may be required to provide better approximation of the hinges with the alignment of the leg.

23. Apply the thigh bars parallel with the femur using a 4-inch roll of plaster (Fig. 15). Fill in the incongruities between the bars and the hardened cylinder with wads of wet plaster. Apply another 3 or 4-inch plaster roll and continue to fill the incongruities by twisting the roll about the hinge arms (Fig. 16). *Mold well* (Fig. 17).

24. Align the hinge arms to the lower leg. Bending irons may be required to allow better approximation to the configuration of the leg (Fig. 18).

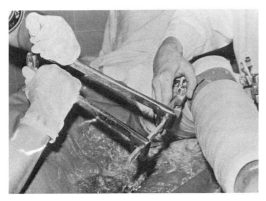

Figure 18.

25. Apply the leg hinges using a 4-inch roll of plaster following the technique described in Step 23 (Fig. 19).

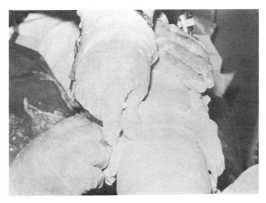

Figure 19.

26. If three persons are available to apply the hinges, one can maintain the position of the bars of the hinges; one can apply the bars to the thigh cylinder; one can apply the bars to the lower leg cylinder.

27. Pad the knee area of the medial hinge to prevent contact with the other leg which could produce bruising.

28. Determine radiographically the position of the hinges relative to the joint.

29. Issue the patient/parent an Allen wrench and instruct in screw adjustment.

30. Adjust the extension screws clockwise and the desubluxation screws counterclockwise. Indicate on the cast the direction in which to turn the screws (Fig. 20). Adjustment should be made daily to pain tolerance. The hinges may be loosened several times during the day to allow the knee to flex through the available arc of motion. The static corrective forces should then be resumed. Two and one-half degrees of extension result from each turn of the proximal screws; the desubluxation screws move about $1/16$ inch with each counterclockwise turn.

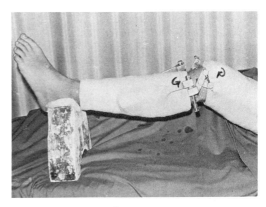

Figure 20.

31. Caution the patient/parent to observe any signs of skin irritation or numbness or tingling in the foot or leg. Ordinarily these symptoms can be relieved by adjusting the screws to allow the knee to flex for a few minutes. Persistent evidence of skin or neurovascular impairment may necessitate cast removal. Knee and hinge position should be checked radiographically.

32. Encourage walking in the cast with or without crutches.

33. When the hinge cast is removed, repeat radiographs and joint motion measurements are taken. An anterior opened-thigh cast is applied to maintain the correction.

APPENDIX 5
MEDICAL AND DENTAL HISTORY
FOR HEMOPHILIACS

Date _____
Birthdate _____

Name _____
Address _____
Telephone _____
Hematologist _____ Hospital _____
Former dentist and location _____
_____
Referred By _____

HEMOPHILIA HISTORY

Type _____
Severity _____
Have your received plasma or concentrates in the past? _____
Father's family (history of hemophilia) _____
_____
Mother's family (history of hemophilia) _____
_____
Siblings affected _____
_____
_____
Are you on a home-care program? _____
Most recent hospitalization and reason _____
_____
_____
Most common problem _____
_____
_____

MEDICAL HISTORY

General statement of health _____
_____
Allergy or drug reactions _____
_____
Are you being treated for anything except hemophilia at present? _____

174

Have you ever had any of the following: (Circle any "yes")
    Rheumatic fever
    Heart trouble
    Tonsillitis (Strep throat)
    Allergy
    Brain injury
    Tuberculosis
    Epilepsy
    Diabetes
    Asthma
    Tumors, growths, or cancer
    Radiation treatment
    Hepatitis

DENTAL HISTORY

Reason for present dental visit _____
_____
Last dental exam _____
Previous reaction to dental treatment _____
_____
Previous extractions _____
_____
Complications with oral bleeding _____
_____
Dental age _____
Appliances present _____
Habits: Swallowing _____ Thumb sucking _____ Mouth breather _____
                       Tongue thrusting _____ Other _____

PRESENT ORAL CONDITION

Extraoral Findings

Facial skin _____
Saliva and salivary glands _____
Jaws _____ T.M.J. _____
Lips _____ Cheeks _____

Intraoral Findings

Floor of mouth _____ Tongue _____
Hard palate _____ Throat _____
Breath _____

Periodontal Structures

Gingival color and texture _____
Hemorrhage _____ _____ Calculus _____
Oral hygiene _____ Brushing frequency _____
Dentifrice _____ Brush _____

DENTAL DIAGNOSIS

Chart (See dental chart)
Orthodontic needs _____

Previous treatment _____

Pulpal therapy _____

Space lost _____
Supernumerary _____ Congenitally missing _____
Extracted _____
Retained root tips _____

TREATMENT PLAN AND PROGNOSIS

Restorations _____

Prevention recommended _____

Home care instruction _____
Nutrition and diet _____
Additional recommendations:

_____
(Resident)

_____
(Staff)

APPENDIX 6

VISUAL DOCUMENTATION

Alfred Benjamin

Routine photographs are used to illustrate the condition of each new patient registered at the Center. Anterior, lateral, and posterior full body views are taken as well as those portions of the body with particular deformity or unusual findings. These views are repeated periodically on selected patients who show changes in their condition over a period of time. Photographic records are made of a patient's progress before and after treatment such as physical or occupational therapy, casting or splinting, and surgery. Motion pictures are used to record gait patterns as well as other functional activities and any alterations made in the pattern following treatment.

Special photographic techniques include infrared photographs and liquid crystal thermography. Infrared techniques aid in the visualization of the extent of a relatively superficial hemorrhage. Infrared color film is used with Number 12 and Number 20 blue filters. Kodachrome 64 film is used for cholesteric liquid crystal photography. The skin area is prepared with a quick-drying, water-soluble, black solution which dries within two to three minutes. Then, the colorless liquid crystals are sprayed upon the prepared black area. This area shows vivid color patterns in shades of red, yellow, green, and blue. Blue indicates the highest temperature range, while green, yellow, and red indicate progressively cooler ranges. The black base is visible on photographs when the body temperature exceeds the range of the liquid crystals. From this display of the gradations of localized temperature, liquid crystals have been found to be useful in diagnosis. Cholesteric liquid crystal photographs can delineate affected areas as shown in Figures 1 and 2.

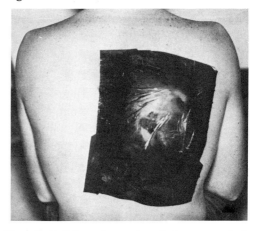

Figure 1. Soft tissue hemorrhage before concentrate administration. Increased surface temperature outlining hematoma is shown by light area.

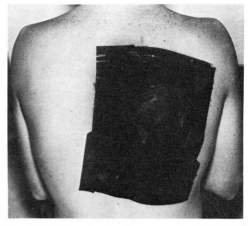

Figure 2. Thirty minutes after concentrate infusion. Note reduced temperature.

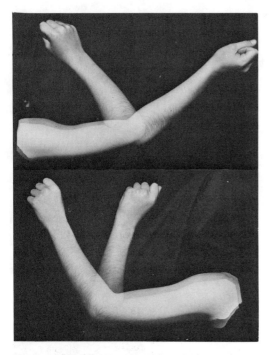

Figure 3. Bilateral elbow restriction: *top,* right arm; *bottom,* left arm.

Range of joint motion is demonstrated by double exposure methods. A camera without double exposure prevention is used; the flash is activated before the motion begins and again at the completion of the motion. Figure 3 illustrates bilateral elbow restriction. Figure 4 shows marked knee limitation and Figure 5 shows nearly normal knee motion.

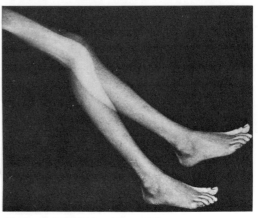

Figure 4. Marked limitation of knee motion.

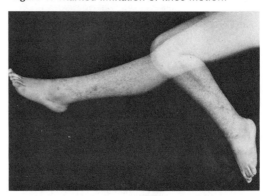

Figure 5. Almost normal knee motion.

INDEX